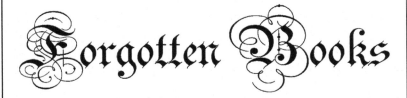
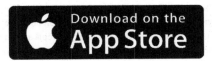

ISBN 978-1-330-33231-3
PIBN 10030322

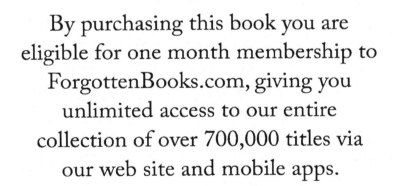

English
Français
Deutsche
Italiano
Español
Português

www.forgottenbooks.com

Mythology Photography **Fiction**
Fishing Christianity **Art** Cooking
Essays Buddhism Freemasonry
Medicine **Biology** Music **Ancient**
Egypt Evolution Carpentry Physics
Dance Geology **Mathematics** Fitness
Shakespeare **Folklore** Yoga Marketing
Confidence Immortality Biographies
Poetry **Psychology** Witchcraft
Electronics Chemistry History **Law**
Accounting **Philosophy** Anthropology
Alchemy Drama Quantum Mechanics
Atheism Sexual Health **Ancient History**
Entrepreneurship Languages Sport
Paleontology Needlework Islam
Metaphysics Investment Archaeology
Parenting Statistics Criminology
Motivational

ORAL ABSCESSES

BY

KURT H. THOMA, D.M.D.

LECTURER ON ORAL HISTOLOGY AND PATHOLOGY AND MEMBER OF THE RESEARCH
DEPARTMENT OF HARVARD UNIVERSITY DENTAL SCHOOL

INSTRUCTOR IN DENTAL ANATOMY, HARVARD MEDICAL SCHOOL
ORAL SURGEON TO THE ROBERT B. BRIGHAM HOSPITAL
VISITING DENTAL SURGEON TO THE LONG ISLAND HOSPITAL
CONSULTING ORAL SURGEON TO THE BOSTON DISPENSARY

BOSTON
RITTER & COMPANY
1916

AUTHOR OF

ORAL ANAESTHESIA

———

LOCAL ANAESTHESIA
IN THE ORAL CAVITY, FOR THE
DIFFERENT BRANCHES
OF DENTISTRY

INTRODUCTION

THE important discovery that septic lesions in the mouth may be foci or primary causes of many acute or chronic diseases of systemic nature has brought about great changes in the relationship between dentistry and medicine. The teeth, which formerly were regarded as organs totally apart from the rest of the body, are now considered as one of the most important gateways through which disease may enter. The dentist who originally held it his duty mechanically to repair diseased or lost dental tissue is now confronted with a problem the vitality of which, if he has a sincere interest in the health of his patients and in the development of his profession, demands a new study of the septic conditions of the mouth.

This book is intended for the practicing dentist as well as for the student. It aims to give a clear understanding of the pathology, treatment, and prevention of oral lesions, and to familiarize the student with the recognition and nature of certain infectious diseases which may be caused by them.

The practicing physician will also find this book of interest. In the search for the primary or secondary foci of systemic diseases he often has occasion to look into the condition of the oral cavity, as it stands out as an important entrance for disease, although it has been until recently neglected as such.

This volume has been written with a view to establishing a correct relationship between the condition of the oral cavity and the health of the patient, and also in the hope that a clear presentation may lead to a more general understanding of this new field.

The author wishes to express his sincere thanks to those of his friends who have aided him in bringing his book before the profession. He wishes especially to express his indebtedness to Dr. T. B. Hartzel for his kind assistance in furnishing colored microphotographs of lesions produced experimentally in the rabbit; to Dr. L. B. Morrison, of the Robert B. Brigham Hospital, for his competent assistance in radiography of hospital cases; to Dr. William *P.* Cooke, for furnishing radiographs; to Dr. W. H. *P*otter, for his examination chart; and to Dean Eugene H. Smith, of the Harvard Dental School, for photographs of models of two cases showing the results of judicious extraction of decayed teeth in children. In connection with the more detailed compilation of the various parts of this volume, the author wishes to thank Miss Herford, for her efficient work in delineation, and Mr. John W. Cooke, for his aid in the preparation of the manuscript.

KURT H. THOMA, D.M.D.

43 BAY STATE ROAD,
    BOSTON, MASSACHUSETTS.
        July 3, 1916.

CONTENTS

CHAPTER I

THE PHENOMENA OF INFECTION

To understand intelligently and fully appreciate the pathology, bacteriology, and treatment of oral abscesses and their secondary manifestations it is well to study first the phenomena of infection generally. The investigations made by Vaughan and Ehrlich and others throw new light on many of these questions. They solved problems of greatest interest which formerly were only vaguely understood. For investigations on focal infection we are indebted especially to Rosenow and Billings. It is my privilege to use freely in this chapter the statements of these authorities.

In all infectious processes there are two principal factors: the infective virus and the body cell. Besides these there is to be considered the environment in which the infection takes place, the unorganized fluids of the body.

THE INFECTIVE VIRUS

The infective virus may be a particular protein and physically different from the medium in which it exists, so that its substance and form can be recognized with the aid of the microscope. This we call a microörganism. It may, on the other hand, be a semi or wholly fluid protein, not sufficiently differentiated from the medium to render it recognizable even with the most delicate microscope. Many such proteins pass through the finest porcelain filters and cannot be deposited even by the centrifuge from the fluids in which they exist.

According to Vaughan, a living protein can be solid, semi-solid, gelatinous, or liquid, but need not be of a form

which our limited senses are capable of recognizing, even
when aided by the most perfect lens. It is capable of
growth and reproduction, and in order to do this it must
assimilate and eliminate. It can only procure this nourishment from material which is within its reach.

A bacteria or another infective virus is, therefore, only
able to live if it can split its surrounding media into
groups which fit into the molecular structure of its cell.
Therefore organisms which can make use of the proteins
of the body in which they live are pathogenic for their
host. If they cannot make use of the substances they
live in they cannot cause an infection.

BACTERIAL FERMENTS   The agents in an organism which prepare
the food for assimilation are called fer-
ments. They are of analytic and synthetic
natures. We also speak of intracellular and extracellular
ferments.

Extracellular Ferments. Extracellular ferments pass
out of the cell and diffuse more or less widely through the
medium which surrounds it. They are of analytic nature,
rendering soluble the proteins of the medium, and the
complex molecules are broken down into simpler structures, some of which can be assimilated, while others
remain as protein poison. The activity of the extracellular ferments is easily affected by modifications in the
medium through which they diffuse. Species of animals,
peculiarities of individuals, slight changes of temperature, or changes in the tissue cause variations in the
growth and multiplication of the bacteria. Hence it is
that one kind of organism grows slowly under unfavorable
conditions, causing chronic disease, while the same bacteria under favorable conditions may cause violent acute
attacks.

Intracellular Ferments. The intracellular ferments
remain in the cell in which they are elaborated and are
in general nondiffusible. They bear a wider variation
in temperature and are not so easily influenced by variations of the composition of the medium in which they
exist. While the extracellular ferments prepare the pro-

teins so that they can be absorbed by the cell, it is left to the intracellular ferments to construct the molecules into the specific proteins which can be assimilated or built into the structure of the cells.

TOXINS *Extracellular Toxin.* Besides these ferments which are necessary to maintain life certain bacteria elaborate another excretion. This is a soluble extracellular substance known as toxin. It is also probably a ferment or a closely allied body. A remarkable characteristic of the toxins is that they are highly specific in their properties and have the power to stimulate the production of antibodies in the infected body. These antibodies are called antitoxins and are also specific. Antitoxin of diphtheria protects only against diphtheria toxin and not against that of any other organism. The number of bacteria-producing toxins, in large quantities at any rate, is small; the diphtheria and tetanus bacilli are good examples of toxin-producing bacteria.

THE BODY CELL

The cells of the body also have ferments, as just described. There is no living organism which does not produce its ferment, and all ferments are produced by living organisms. The preparation of food for assimilation is due to ferment action.

FERMENTS OF THE BODY CELL The ferments of the body cell also work analytically and synthetically. They are of extracellular and intracellular natures. Their primary function is to supply the cells which elaborate them with food. In doing this they also protect the cells to which they belong by destroying the harmful bodies both particulate and formless. They are, however, of a specific nature. While the ferments of the body cells of one animal may digest one or more bacterial proteins, they may be unable to break down the proteins of certain other infectious organisms. Another animal, under the same general conditions, may resist the latter organism, but prove incapable of combating the former. If they are able to break down the bacterial proteins these are destroyed and the animal will resist disease.

THE PHAGOCYTES Some cells not only destroy invading organisms by their extracellular ferments, as just described, but even engulf entire bodies of bacteria and dispose of protein poisons, digesting them by the action of their intracellular ferments. Cells with such functions are the wandering leucocytes, lymphocytes, plasma cells, as well as fixed endothelial and connective tissue cells.

TWO BIOLOGI-CAL LAWS Vaughan* formulated the following biological laws which well describe the phenomena of infection.

1. If the body cells are permeated or come in contact with a foreign protein (bacteria), the former elaborates a specific ferment by which the latter are destroyed.

2. If the body cells are attacked by destructive ferments (toxins), the former form anti-ferments (antitoxins) which have the office of neutralizing the ferments to protect the body cells.

PROTECTIVE DEFENCES OF THE BODY

The body cells of the host attempt in the manner described to resist the growth and multiplication of the foreign proteins: this growth constitutes infection. The

RESISTANCE resistance in an animal or a person has been found to be greater at one time and diminished at another. In youth the resistance is smaller than in old age.

Decrease of Resistance. The proteolytic action of the body cells, which checks the progress of infection, can be greatly decreased or removed by any cause which lowers the general or local vitality of the tissue. Among these belong hunger and starvation, bad ventilation, overexertion, exposure to cold, acute or chronic diseases, and focal infection. Local affections such as injury, tissue changes

---

* *See* Bibliography.

from disease, the presence of foreign bodies, and the interference with the circulation of the blood also tend to lessen the vitality.

Increase of Resistance. All conditions which are favorable to the health of the body increase its resistance and render the tissue cells more able to overcome the infection. Healthy food, beneficial exercise, and good circulation, fresh air and all prophylactic means further an increase in the resisting power of the body. The treatment of disease and the careful search for and surgical removal of chronic foci, from which protein poison or toxins are absorbed, will also remove causes which sap the vitality of the individual and lower the resistance against new infections.

BACTERIAL IMMUNITY   *Natural Immunity.* Natural immunity is due either to the fact that bacteria are unable to feed upon the proteins of the body and therefore cannot live, or because they are destroyed by the specific ferment, formed as a protective measure by the body cells. There are germicidal agents found dissolved in the plasma as well as in the serum. These are probably extracellular ferments, while similar agents are found in these cells themselves, which are probably intracellular ferments. The first act directly on protein organisms if they are contained in the plasma or blood serum; the latter act only after these organisms have permeated into the body cells which produce them. Cells which have such functions in a marked degree are called phagocytes.

Acquired Immunity. Immunity is acquired either by disease or by therapeutic measures.

Immunity which is due to recovery from an infection is the result of the development in the body, during the course of infection, of a specific ferment which on renewed exposures immediately destroys the infection.

Immunity established by vaccination is similar to that induced by an attack of the disease. A vaccine is the same protein that causes the disease. It is, however,

modified by passage through animals, by growth at high
temperature, or by killing the bacteria by heat, so that
it does not induce the disease but yet it must be so little
altered that it will stimulate the body cells to form a
specific ferment which will promptly on exposure destroy
the infecting agent.   This process also is called "protein
sensitization."

TOXIN IMMUNITY To understand toxin immunity it is necessary to first understand toxin activity.   The
toxin, which is produced only by a small
number of bacteria, is a soluble and diffusible ferment.
It splits up the proteins of the body, setting free the
protein poison.   The body cells of animals are stimulated
by this to produce an antitoxin which neutralizes the
toxin and prevents its cleavage action.   The antitoxin
does not destroy the foreign proteins, as do the proteolytic
ferments of the body cells, but only prevents the action
of the elaborated toxin.

Antitoxin for therapeutic purposes can be produced by
injecting the toxin, gained by injecting a very virulent
culture in broth, into an animal, usually a young horse.
The serum of the horse then contains the antitoxin.   Antitoxin is rather a preventive than a cure.   It is much
more active if given before or in the very beginning of
the infection.   The immunity procured with serum containing antitoxin is but temporary.

THE PROCESS OF INFECTION

*P*athogenic proteins entering the body feed upon man's
proteins, and they convert the body proteins into bac-
INCUBATION terial proteins by their digestive ferments.
They grow and multiply rapidly.   This
is essentially a process of building up, as no poisonous
protein is liberated and the process goes on without any
recognizable disturbance in the health of the body.   We
call this stage of infection the period of incubation.   During this period the body cells do not resist the growth
and multiplication of the foreign protein.

During the period of incubation the body cells are being prepared for their combat with the foreign proteins.

SENSITIZA-TION From the action of the foreign protein on the body cell we note the development in the latter of a specific proteolytic ferment, a new function. This process we call protein sensitization. It is a process of distinction of the invading organisms. The new ferment digests the invading proteins, setting free the protein poison.

PROTEIN POISON (*Intracellular Toxin*) *caused by bacterial destruction.* After the body cells have been sensitized the specific ferment which is formed starts at once to break down the bacterial cells. This, however, does not mean that the analytic process of the bacteria is stopped at this moment; on the contrary the constructive action of the bacterial ferments continues, the invading organisms still grow and multiply but the process of destruction is going on at the same time. A fight for supremacy ensues between the invading organisms by their fermentive action of bacterial construction and the defending body cells by their destructive action of their newly-formed proteolytic ferments. All bacteria contain an intracellular poison which is a group in the protein molecule and is neutralized in most organisms by combination with nonpoisonous groups. Therefore such proteins have no action until they undergo molecular disruption. It is the action of the proteolytic ferments which splits the molecules of the invading proteins, setting free the protein poison (intracellular toxin) which makes the symptoms of the disease appear. Protein poison is not a true toxin, although the term toxin is loosely applied to all poisons of infectious origin. It is formed during all processes of infection, while true toxin, as we have already seen, is a special ferment characteristic of certain bacteria. Protein poison is produced by destruction of the bacterial proteins, is not affected by heat and does not excite the formation of an antibody and differs probably in quality with the variety of the bacteria.

Protein Poison Caused by Bacterial Metabolism from the Body Cells. It has already been described how bacteria split by their extracellular ferments the surrounding media of their host. From the newly-formed structures some are absorbed and others remain as protein poison. The intracellular ferments split again into molecules which are assimilated and built into the structure of the cell, and substances which are excreted. These by-products of extracellular and intracellular bacterial metabolism may be harmless or may be important protein poisons. Their nature depends upon the special action of the ferment as well as the quality of the media of the host in which the bacteria grow.

The action of the bacterial ferments. The action of the bacterial ferments is of greatly varied nature. There are proteolytic ferments, hemolysin,. nuclease, lab-ferment, lipase, diastatic ferments, invertase, pectase, gelase, oxydase and katalase.

The Influence of the Medium. There is usually a substance which the bacteria are able to digest particularly easily, but if this is not present they will attack harder and less accessible material. The chemical make-up of the medium naturally has a great deal to do with the result and with the by-products of bacterial metabolism.

By-products of Bacterial Metabolism. The by-products of the extra- and intracellular ferment action of the bacteria are almost always relatively strong poisons to the host. Various colored pigments are formed which have not been studied very much. From nitrogenized bodies, or proteid substances which constitute the greater proportion of animal tissue, there are formed complicated protein poisons, ammonia, ptomaines, alkalies, hydrogen sulphid, aromatics (Indol, Skatol, Phenol, Tyrosin) and gases such as Nitrogen. From carbohydrates and animal fats there are formed acids (lactic acid, Formic acid, acetic acid, butyric acid) and gases (carbon dioxide, Nitrogen, methane, Hydrogen).

This process of bacterial action is a decomposition, resulting in various combinations of the by-products of the metabolism. These by-products can almost always be recognized by the sense of smell and it is small wonder that such substances if absorbed into the system cause diseases of all kinds.

Toxin. Toxin is a term which is clinically applied in a loose manner to any poisonous substances formed during the process of infection. It includes in this sense ferments, extra- and intracellular toxin, and any protein poison produced by the process of bacterial metabolism.

In its strict sense the term toxin is, as we have already seen, applied only to the specific extracellular bacterial poisons, as these alone cause the body cells to produce antitoxins.

CLINICAL PICTURE OF THE INFECTION

The clinical picture and course of the infection depend upon several factors.

Influence of Quantity in Infection. The number of pathogenic organisms introduced into the body plays a great rôle. A small number of bacteria may die, while from a large number a certain amount is sure to survive and cause disease.

Influence of Bacterial Growth on Infection. Bacteria differ as to the rapidity with which they grow. This depends mostly upon the conditions they find; if the body proteins are easily digested they grow rapidly but if they can make use of the proteins of their host only with difficulty and if the circumstances under which they have to grow are unfavorable, as exclusion of oxygen for aerobic bacteria, the growth and multiplication is slow. This also has its reaction upon the body cells. If the infective virus multiplies rapidly, sensitization of the body cells is general and starts early. If the infecting organism finds less favorable conditions for its growth it multiplies slowly and the body cells are sensitized locally.

Influence of Virulence in Infection. With bacteria whose virulence is great, disease will be produced quickly by a small number of bacteria, while a very large number is necessary if the bacteria is of the low virulent type.

Acute and Chronic Infection. If the pathogenic organisms enter the body in large number, increase rapidly, or are highly virulent, and sensitization of the body cells therefore is marked, starts early and is general, the developing disease is acute. If only few organisms invade the body, or if the infecting organisms multiply slowly and find unfavorable conditions, if sensitization of the body cells is mild and only local, the disease takes a chronic course.

LOCAL INFECTION

If the infecting virus and the sensitization of the body cells is limited to a certain part of the body, we call the infection local.

LOCAL EFFECTS The effect of the toxins (protein poisons) upon the body cells gives rise to various kinds of inflammation such as serous, fibrinous, purulent, necrotic, gangrenous or proliferative. Serous exudations into the subcutaneous tissue follow certain bacterial infections in certain tissues, while the same or other bacteria cause purulent inflammation in other tissues or under other conditions.

GENERAL EFFECTS *Fever.* Heat is produced during the processes of infection from the following sources: (1) from the unaccustomed stimulation and consequent increased activity of the cells which supply the ferments; (2) from the cleavage of the foreign protein; and (3) from the reaction between the proteolytic ferment of the body cells and the foreign proteins, especially if active and virulent poison is liberated. Fever must therefore be regarded as a beneficent process although it often leads to disaster, especially if the reaction takes place with great rapidity. The temperature is the most delicate test of the severity of the inflammation.

Changes in the Blood. The microbian proteins almost always produce an increase in the number of leucocytes and a decrease in the amount of protein. The red blood cells are sometimes directly injured by some of the bacterial substances.

GENERAL INFECTION

If the infective virus is distributed widely through the whole body and if sensitization of the tissue cells is general, we speak of general infection. Today we know that infections are never entirely localized and that there is always absorption of bacteria or of the toxins formed by the infectious process.

TOXEMIA The result from absorption of bacterial toxins (either true toxins or toxins of bacterial metabolism) varies according to the quality and amount absorbed. If the system is flooded by large amounts, so that there are marked symptoms of intoxication, we have the picture of acute toxemia. The process, however, may go on for years without causing gross symptoms, and we have a chronic toxemia which often causes physical discomfort and mental depression.

BACTEREMIA If the bacteria are absorbed in quantity into the blood and multiply, we have an acute general infection called septicemia, which is of most severe character, resulting often in death.

Frequently, however, we find conditions when bacteria are not potent enough to cause gross symptoms of infection, although they actually wear out the cells, whose duty it is to combat and kill them, thus lowering the resistance of the body.

METASTASIS The presence of bacteria or toxins in the blood and tissue fluid may cause new infections or diseased conditions in other parts of the body, which are either predisposed by lowered resistance or which have a special affinity for the injurious agent.

SECONDARY OR TRANSPORTED INFECTIONS

Billings says: *"The knowledge of the principle of secondary infection is of importance for preventive as well as therapeutic treatment. The recognition and the removal of the focus is imperative to prevent secondary disease and is demanded as a fundamental principle to stop the progression of ill-health."*

It has just been shown that bacteria and toxins are absorbed from local infections into the blood and that new infections occur at remote parts of the body. This is called secondary or transported infection, a process which has been discovered only recently but which is of frequent occurrence.

THE FOCUS The focus may be found in any part of the body and may be an acute or chronic local infection. Foci are sometimes apparent, but often only recognized after careful examination by the specialist. They may be in the nose and adjacent sinuses, the oral cavity, the throat, the alimentary canal, or the genitourinary system.

CHANNELS OF ABSORPTION Bacteria and their products are absorbed through two channels, the blood and the lymph system. They are carried into the blood by passive entrance through the stomata of the capillary walls, by growth of the bacteria through walls of the vessels, and by carriage into the blood by leucocytes. They also may reach the blood by the way of the lymph vessels after their transmission through the lymph glands. The deeper the infection is seated in the tissue, and the greater the pressure of the accumulated bacterial products, the larger is the amount of absorption. Also the tissue in which the infection occurs is of importance. Mucous membrane absorbs easily. An abscess enclosed by bone gives no chance for infiltration or extension; therefore the pressure is great and the bacterial products are absorbed readily. If there is a sinus the pressure is decreased and the amount of absorption is diminished. When abscesses or other lesions discharge their exudates into the mouth, they reach different parts of the alimentary canal where a new focus may be formed, especially if the pus supply is long continued. But secondary lesions may in turn also become foci for further and more general infection. Such conditions must not be mistaken for the primary cause of the focal disease, but they should be removed so that they will not serve to further prolong and intensify the disease. (Billings.)

ORAL FOCI   Oral foci may cause secondary infections via the capillary or lymph system. Absorption is most likely to be caused by blind, acute, or chronic abscesses, but occurs also from pyorrhoea pockets, diseased gums, and other lesions of the mucous membrane. But infection may also occur by pus discharging into the oral cavity, as in pyorrhoea, and suppurative gingivitis caused by poorly fitted crowns and bridges, and in alveolar abscesses with sinus; the result then is mostly a local infection such as stomatitis, pharyngitis, or an infection of the alimentary canal, as septic gastritis, enteritis, or appendicitis. But if the surface immunity of the digestive tract is overcome, the alimentary canal will become a new focus, bacteria being absorbed, causing further secondary infection.

Oral abscesses, especially of the unsuspected chronic type, are in these days of overdentistried teeth a common infection and are of greatest importance in the diagnosis and treatment of secondary disease. The unsuspecting and deceived individual is usually not aware of the menace which has undermined his health or is ready to cause the most terrible chronic diseases if the conditions for secondary infections are right.

SECONDARY MANIFESTATIONS   The part of the body affected and the disease produced by absorbed toxins and bacteria depends upon several factors. The different toxins have special affinities for a certain tissue. The varieties of bacteria have preferences to grow in certain tissues and even strains of a certain class of bacteria have a predilection of the place in which they may accumulate. Some forms of streptococci grow only in conditions with abundant oxygen supply (endocarditis), while others prefer places of decreased oxygen tension (arthritis). The part of the body in which they start a secondary infection is often predisposed by traumatic injury or lowered resistance from other reasons.

A place which is liable to become affected by secondary disease may at other times be the seat of the focus, while lesions which usually are primary infections can be caused by transported or secondary infection. Alveolar abscesses are almost always primary lesions whether they are the cause of secondary disease or not, but occasionally abscess formation starts on devitalized teeth, with perfect root-canal fillings from haematogenous infection, due to diseased tonsils or some other focus.

PLATE I

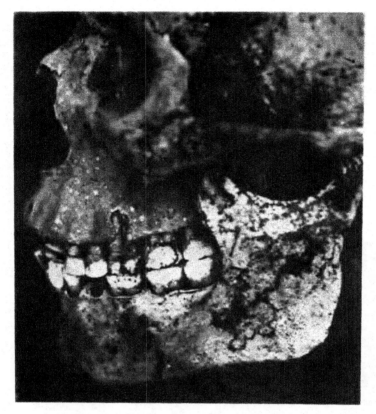

FIG. 1.—Predynastic Egyptian Skull from Upper Egypt. shows loss of bone due to abscess condition on the buccal roots of the upper first molar.   The pulp in this tooth was exposed from abrasion.

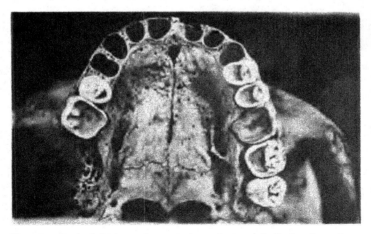

FIG. 2.—Occlusial view of upper jaw of same skull showing abrasion of the teeth and the exposed pulp chamber of the first molar.

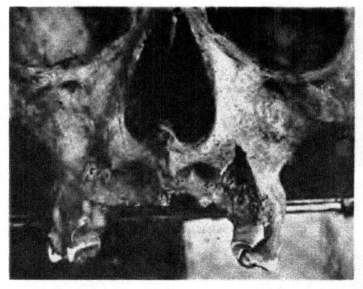

FIG. 3.—Prehistoric Peruvian skull from the cave Huaricauc. There is a great deal of bone lost in the upper incisor region from acute abscess condition.

CHAPTER II

HISTORY AND VARIETIES OF ORAL ABSCESSES

HISTORY Abscesses of the teeth are known to have occurred centuries ago. We find their bone destructive processes both about the jaws of ancient civilized people such as the Egyptians, as well as in ancient native tribes.

The older literature knows only the alveolar abscess with acute symptoms of calor, dolor, rudor, and tumor, while the discharge of pus from sinuses on the gum which gave the patient no discomfort was an obscure quantity neglected by the dentist who then considered it his duty only to relieve pain and plug cavities. Later this condition was considered the termination of the acute alveolar abscess which did not yield to treatment. It was called chronic alveolar abscess.

Abscess sacks found adhering to extracted roots or teeth furthered the knowledge of the pathology of the dental abscesses, and in cases where neither the gum nor the tooth showed any sign of suppurating condition, the term "blind abscess" was applied. The blind abscess usually gave no apparent discomfort and therefore was classified with the chonic abscess. At that time, teeth with diseased pulps were either neglected by the patient, or if treatment and relief of pain was sought, extracted. But when the value of the teeth for mastication became better understood, men set out to preach the saving of teeth, and methods were invented to treat the pulpless teeth. I do not believe that the fathers of conservative dentistry meant to convey the meaning of the doctrine which became popular. It is not reasonable to try to save every tooth, no matter how diseased it is and how inaccessible the root-canals may be. But it was expected of every dentist that his greatest aim should be to save all teeth and that it showed lack of ability to be obliged to sacrifice a tooth. On account of the difficulty of root-canal operations and the obscurity of the achievement, the results frequently were poor, even if careful technique were employed, and miserable if carelessly incompetent. Because recommendation of extraction was looked upon with disfavor, the many overdentistried teeth with incomplete root-canal work were left in the mouth. The resulting condition was apparently normal. There was no discomfort or perhaps only slight grumbling sensations, overlooked by dentist and patient.

Not until the X-rays were applied for diagnosis in dentistry have we discovered the true condition of such teeth, and since the progressive dentist secures the services of the dental radiologist, or has an X-ray machine of his own, we stand before the grave fact that most pulpless teeth are the cause of chronic inflammatory processes in the alveolar process of the maxillary and mandibular bone, which give no trouble or only the slightest local symptoms, but are the cause of much ill-health and disease.

CLASSIFICA-TION Oral abscesses are best divided into three classes according to their etiological factors:

1. Alveolar abscesses caused by diseases of the dental pulp.

2. Alveolar abscesses due to other causes than diseases of the dental pulp.

3. Abscesses of the tongue, salivary glands, and ducts.

The first class is by far the most important one; it includes acute alveolar abscesses caused usually by acute diseases of the pulp and the chronic alveolar abscesses which are so commonly found on pulpless teeth. It has been estimated that these are found in the mouth of a large percentage of the population of the United States. In the Robert B. Brigham Hospital, where the only patients are those who suffer from chronic diseases, I found such abscesses in eighty-eight per cent. of the patients examined. The second class includes abscesses caused by pyorrhoea, infection of the gums, and impacted and unerupted teeth. These are by far less frequent than the previous group.

In the third class we have conditions which are of rather rare occurrence and are frequently secondary to diseases of the teeth. However, abscesses may occur on the tongue and in the salivary glands and in ducts, which are due to various other causes.

CHAPTER III

PATHOLOGICAL DEVELOPMENT OF ALVE-OLAR ABSCESSES CAUSED BY DIS-EASES OF THE DENTAL PULP

VARIETIES Generally alveolar abscesses due to dis-eases of the pulp have been divided into two classes: the acute and the chronic condition. This division is selected, according to the large or small amount of discomfort the patient experiences, that is, according to the symptoms, without considering either the etiology, the histopathological picture, or the termination of the disease. We know that the acute alveolar abscess if not cured will terminate in the chronic form, but some of the so-called "chronic" forms occur without passing through the acute stage. As a matter of fact, since only a very small percentage of chronic abscesses have ever started with symptoms of discomfort, the classification of "acute" and "chronic" is therefore not scientifically correct. A closer study of the pathological stages shows that *the acute abscess involves a process of destruction* while the so-called *chronic abscess is a process of inflammatory new growth*. This proliferating new growth is of a more or less circumscribed character, while the acute condition of destruction is of a diffuse nature, spreading into the adjacent parts.

I shall therefore distinguish two varieties of alveolar abscesses due to diseases of the dental pulp. Both represent a progressive chain of pathological changes, the first of a destructive, the second of a constructive, nature.

1. *Acute Periodontitis and its sequels*—or changes of destructive nature beginning with acute periodontitis,

PLATE III

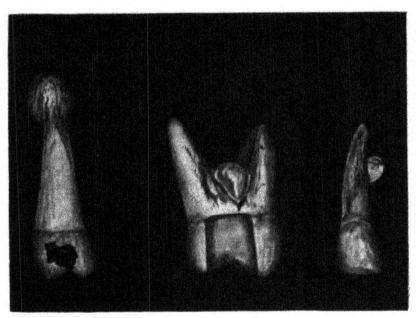

FIG. 4.—Bicuspid with apical abscess.   Incisor with lateral abscess.
Molar with inter-radial abscess.

culminating in acute alveolar abscess or alveolar parulis, and ending in chronic alveolar abscess and its sequels.

2. *Proliferating Periodontitis and its sequels*—or changes stimulating inflammatory new growth beginning with proliferating periodontitis and resulting in a granuloma.

1. ACUTE PERIODONTITIS AND ITS SEQUELS

DEFINITION Acute periodontitis and its sequels are changes which involve suppurative destruction of the surrounding tissues of the tooth, culminating in a collection of pus in or about the alveolar processes, called alveolar abscess or alveolar parulis.

Acute Apical Periodontitis. The natural outlet from the pulp chamber is the apical foramen, or the apical foramina, and therefore we find these openings the most common mouths of the infection, since they are the natural passages through which infected matter may pass from the dental pulp chamber into the surrounding tissues of the apex of the tooth. The sequel of the acute apical periodontitis is the "apical alveolar abscess."

Acute Interradial Periodontitis. This is inflammation which occurs between the roots of multirooted teeth from decay extending from the diseased dental pulp through the floor of the pulp chamber. Infection by perforation of the floor of the pulp chamber or inner sides of the roots with burr or root canal instruments also gives rise to this condition. Its sequel is the *acute interradial alveolar abscess.*

Acute Lateral Periodontitis. Perforation of and infection through the lateral wall of a tooth by the burr or root-canal instrument gives rise to inflammation of the periodontal membrane, resulting in a lateral alveolar abscess.

ETIOLOGY The diseases of the dental pulp or pulp chamber are responsible for the formation of acute periodontitis, which later develops into the acute alveolar abscess. This condition is always due to a

large invasion of virulent pyogenic bacteria. The causes
of the infection are the following:

Traumatic Injury of a Tooth. Injuries received by
falling or from a blow result in inflammation of the pulp.
The tooth may be fractured in the crown, exposing the
pulp to outside influences, or fractured in the root, exposing it to the irritation caused by the fractured seg-
ments. The hard substances of the tooth are almost
always fractured if traumatic injury occurs, but occasionally this does not take place and pulpitis is then
caused by injury to the tissue in the periapical regions.
The same condition occurs occasionally from the action
of orthodontia appliances, if force has been applied too
abruptly or if the teeth are moved too rapidly. The interference with the circulation of the pulp and the lowered
resistance of the tissue invite hematogenous infection,
which results in suppuration of the tissues involved. In
this way acute periodontitis may result from primary infection of the periapical region or by means of the pulp
if the injury occurred in the crown or side of the root. If
no therapeutic measures interfere, this will develop into
an acute alveolar abscess.

Infection from Adjacent Teeth. Suppuration often
spreads in the cancellous part of the alveolar process
causing acute infection of the periodontal membrane of
adjacent teeth. If the infection occurs in this manner
there is, however, less danger of involvement of the pulp
if it is in good condition. Neighboring teeth are frequently involved to an extent which makes them so loose
that their condition seems hopeless, but the pulp resists
disease in these cases for a long period, and if the cause
is removed in time, the periodontal membrane, the fibres
of which have a wonderful resisting power to destruction,
returns to normal and the tooth regains its firmness in
the jaw. Occasionally, however, especially if drainage
of the abscess is delayed, the pulp becomes infected, resulting in violent suppurating pulpitis.

Infections from Pus Pockets. Pus pockets between
the gum and the tooth are the result of the destruction

PLATE IV

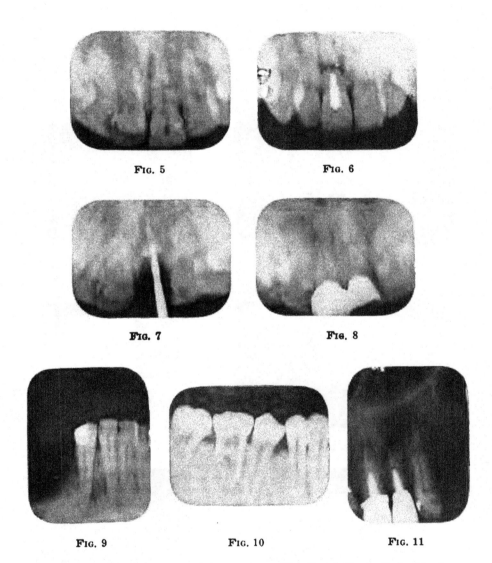

FIG. 5   FIG. 6

FIG. 7   FIG. 8

FIG. 9   FIG. 10   FIG. 11

FIGS. 5 and 6.—Abscess caused by trauma. The tip of the teeth having been fractured.

FIGS. 7 and 8.—Show the treatment of the case Fig. 5. The tooth was extracted and replaced by a porcelain tooth, the root having been carved according to the X-ray picture and attached to the next tooth.

FIGS. 9, 10 and 11.—Show teeth with abscesses which have involved neighboring teeth.

PLATE V

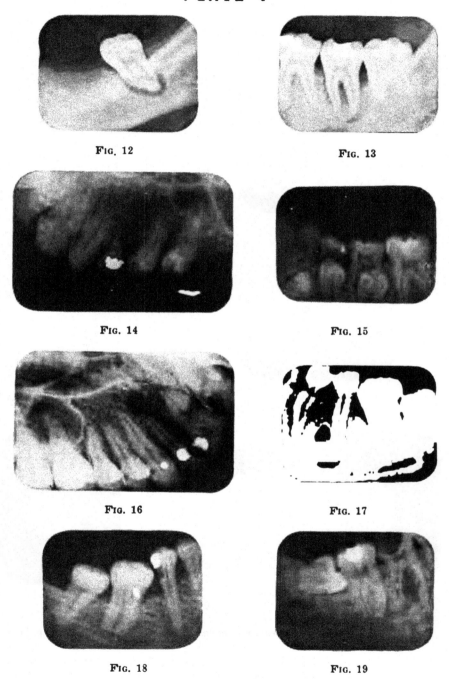

FIG. 12   FIG. 13

FIG. 14   FIG. 15

FIG. 16   FIG. 17

FIG. 18   FIG. 19

FIGS. 12 and 13.—Apical abscesses due to pyorrhea pockets.
FIGS. 14 and 15.—Abscesses from temporary teeth.
FIGS. 16, 17, 18, and 19.—Abscesses due to decay of permanent teeth. In Figures
17 and 18 the decay has started under the filling.

of the alveolar process surrounding the tooth by pyorrhoea alveolaris or of septic descending periodontitis caused by unclean, unsanitary, ill-fitting, evil crowns and bridges as well as irritating fillings. The infection progresses towards the apex, and when it reaches this part, it destroys the blood supply of the pulp, producing septic pulpitis and apical alveolar abscess, which usually discharges through the pocket.

Thermal Shocks Conducted to the Pulp by Large Metal Fillings cause hyperemia of the pulp, and if the irritation is strong enough and continued, it will result in pulpitis, death of the pulp, and alveolar abscess.

Crowned Teeth. Teeth, fitted with entire porcelain or gold crowns, either for purposes of restoration of lost tissue or for bridge work, are often believed to become devitalized because contact with air and with the fluids of the mouth is prevented. It is the author's opinion that this is not the real cause. The latest discovery in dental histology teaches us that the dentin metabolism comes from the dental pulp, while only the metabolism of the adult enamel is dependent on the fluids of the mouth. The metabolism of the dentin of a tooth, which is covered entirely by a crown, is therefore not interfered with. From practical experience we know that a great number of teeth with well-fitted, entire crowns, stay in perfectly healthy condition, while the pulps of others die. Two reasons can be attributed to the death of the pulp in these cases. It may be due to thermal shock, and from the grinding which is necessary to reduce the contour of the tooth. The second reason is decay, which has not been entirely removed, or, which is caused by ill-fitting crowns.

Decay of Deciduous Teeth. Deciduous teeth are very frequently neglected and their office is very vaguely understood by most of the patients. The need of teeth for the purpose of mastication is most important in children because they require more nourishment than the adult to build up their bodies and to resist childhood illnesses. These should perform the function of masti-

cation until the permanent teeth erupt. Their other duty is
to hold the space open and prevent other teeth from mov-
ing forward until the permanent teeth take their place,
in order to prevent malocclusion. This function which
concerns normal occlusion of the permanent teeth is of
greatest importance and should stimulate us to keep these
temporary teeth in good condition so as to prevent their
pulps from becoming diseased. Acute abscesses form
easily on deciduous teeth if the pulp has been infected on
account of the physiological process of bone absorption
caused by the eruption of their successors—and this infection is easily carried into deeper areas; indeed, fistulas
to the face, cervical and submaxillary adenitis caused by
temporary teeth are very frequently found in children.
If the disease has progressed to the stage of an acute
abscess, the question arises whether these teeth should
be extracted with malocclusion as a consequence, or
whether they should be retained with the risk of infection
and its serious possibilities involving the development,
health, and even the life of the patient.

Decay of the Permanent Teeth. Caries of the dentin
if not stopped will progress in the dentinal tubules and
cause suppurative pulpitis before the cavity has reached
the pulp; frequently, however, the cavity extends directly
into the pulp chamber. The same process of infection
develops from decay which has not been entirely removed, before restoring the shape of the tooth by crown
or filling. The pulp may also be infected during the
therapeutic act of excavating a cavity. Even a pulp
exposure of minute size, almost always has suppurative
pulpitis as a consequence, unless it receives the careful
treatment which is called pulp-capping. This treatment
is advisable only in children's teeth, when the root canal
is wide open, which prevents strangulation during the
usually resulting period of hyperemia and mild inflammation. In the cases where the decay forms an opening
into the pulp chamber, the disease very seldom affects
the periapical tissue. The exudates escape through this
outlet, and after the stage of inflammation, the pulp tis-

sue degenerates and frequently becomes hypertrophied, which is a measure of protection. But if suppuration occurs in a tooth with a filling, or where the natural opening becomes stopped up by food or other substances, the infectious matter is forced through the apical foramen and forms an acute alveolar abscess.

Filling of Teeth with Infected Pulps. A tooth with an open root canal and a pulp or part of a pulp in acute inflammatory condition should not be sealed up after the first treatment has been applied, because in doing so we would close the natural outlet through which the products of fermentation and suppuration make their escape; these products would be forced through the apical foramen and infect the periapical tissue. Such treatment is often the result of acute periodontitis and acute alveolar abscess.

Instrumentation. Instruments inserted into septic root canals and root-canal instruments used for cleaning of septic root canals act often as plungers forcing septic material through the apical foramen into the periapical tissue, inoculating directly the periodontal membrane and the bone. Such instruments should therefore not be used until the bacteria have been destroyed by antiseptic drugs. Perforation of the floor of the pulp chamber in multi-rooted teeth or piercing of the sides of a root with a root-canal instrument may also be the cause of acute periodontitis and acute abscess.

Change in Oxygen Tension. Very often a tooth with a diseased pulp is in a quiescent condition until the pulp chamber is opened in order to gain access for treatment. The patient will return the next day with all symptoms of an acute periodontitis, having suffered a great deal of pain during the night. This is due to a change in oxygen tension, and the bacteria which developed only slowly because of lack of oxygen now become extremely active on account of the access of air, causing suppuration which will progress through the apical foramen if the tooth is sealed hermetically after the operation.

COURSE OF THE DISEASE   *Acute Periodontitis.* If bacteria or products of suppuration escape through the apical foramen, the periodontal membrane is first attacked, causing acute apical periodontitis. The swelling of the blood vessels and the serous infiltration enlarges the periodontal membrane and pushes the tooth for a short distance out of the socket. This stage of hyperemia is of short duration. Small particles of pus collect near the apical foramen and soon spread between the fibres of the periodontal membrane, which finally becomes dissolved. A tooth extracted at this stage shows, if the periodontal membrane adheres to the cementum, a red appearance in the apical region. The apical periodontitis may spread over the whole surface of the root and is then called acute total periodontitis.

Acute Alveolar Abscess. The inflammation now involves the linea dura, the compact layer of bone lining the alveolar socket. The bone is destroyed as suppuration progresses and the cavity formed fills with pus. This condition is called acute alveolar abscess.

Alveolar Parulis. The pus which stands more or less under pressure proceeds in the cancellous part of the bone and finds its way through some Haversian canals, penetrating the plate or dense cortical layer surrounding the bone. This stage is sometimes reached in a short time, as quickly as overnight, but at other times, especially in the mandible, it takes four to five days for the pus to burrow to the surface.

Subperiosteal Parulis. The Haversian canals are enlarged and show in dissected skulls as small perforations through which the pus escapes between the bone and periosteum. The periosteum, like the periodontal membrane, is tough and has a considerable resisting quality to destruction. The pus therefore spreads under the periosteum and often accumulates in large quantity, sometimes causing a widely distributed oedematic swelling of the face.

PLATE VI

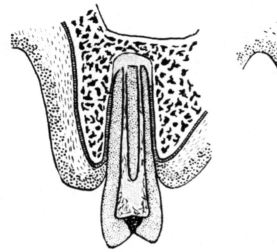

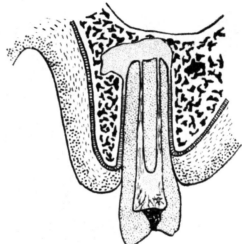

Fɪɢ. 20

Fɪɢ. 21

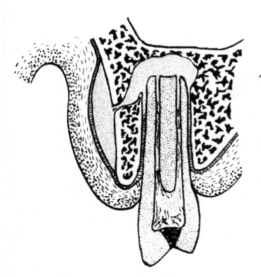

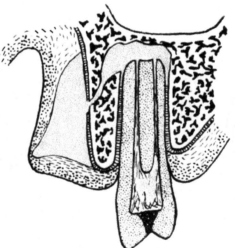

Fɪɢ. 22

Fɪɢ. 23

Fɪɢ. 20.—Acute periodontitis.
Fɪɢ. 21.—Acute abscess.
Fɪɢ. 22.—Subperiostial parulis.
Fɪɢ. 23.—Sub-gingival parulis.

PLATE VII

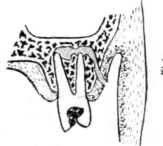
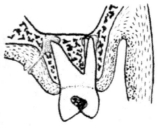
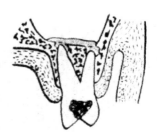

FIG. 24   FIG. 25   FIG. 26

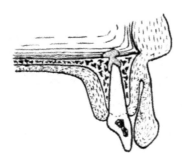
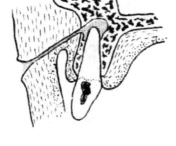

FIG. 27   FIG. 28

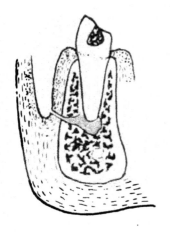
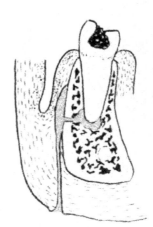
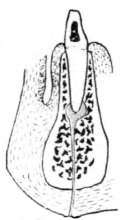
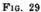

FIG. 29   FIG. 30   FIG. 31

FIG. 24.—Sinus to the gum.
FIG. 25.—Sinus to the palate.
FIG. 26.—Sinus into the antrum.
FIG. 27.—Sinus into the nasal cavity.
FIG. 28.—Sinus to the cheek.
FIG. 29.—Sinus to the gum of the lower jaw.
FIG. 30.—Sinus to the skin of the lower jaw progressing along the outside of the bone.
FIG. 31.—Sinus to the chin.

Subgingival Parulis. If the pus penetrates the periosteum and collects under the gum we speak of a subgingival parulis. This stage is usually reached quickly, but, in other cases, only after the subperiosteal parulis has lasted for a long time. The rate depends on the resistance of the periosteum. The swelling caused by the subgingival parulis is more rounded, while the tumor of the subperiosteal parulis is flat.

Sinus from Acute Alveolar Abscess into the Mouth. If the pressure of the pus at this stage is not relieved by surgical interference, the parulis will come to a point and break through the gum, usually opposite the apex of the root. This passage is called a sinus. The course of the pus, however, is not always so direct. If the periosteum is very resistant and if the pus accumulates in large quantity, it may follow the laws of gravity and least resistance and pierce the periosteum at a place quite remote from its source. Sinuses occur almost always at the buccal or labial part of the gum; palatal sinuses are more rare and usually are derived from the superior incisor teeth and often lead some distance back into the mouth. Sinuses are still more rare at the lingual gum of the lower teeth, from which point the pus usually sinks downwards, involving the tissues of the floor of the mouth.

Sinus from Acute Alveolar Abscess to the Face. If the pus does not readily find an outlet through the gum, it passes along fascias and muscles through submucous and subcutaneous tissue until it reaches the skin of the face. Here it collects in a similar way, as under the gum. It causes a swelling and extends the skin to its limit before it penetrates to the surface. (Fig. 30.) The course of the sinus is often a long and tortuous one. Sinuses to the skin occur especially from severe subperiosteal parulis and are often caused by ignorant application of heat or poultices to the outside of the face to relieve the pain. Sinus to the face from the upper jaw is not very common. If it occurs, the outlet usually is near the malar process, as seen in Fig. 28. In the lower jaw the pus settles more frequently into the tissue, breaking below the lower border of the mandible. The pus has been found to follow the course of muscles, finally finding an outlet on the neck or chest. From the inside of the mouth and from the front teeth the sinus, if it does not find any outlet to the gum, leads almost always to the chin.

Sinus for Acute Alveolar Abscess to the Antrum of Highmore. The roots of the superior bicuspids and molars sometimes extend into the antrum and are covered only by the linea dura of the alveolar socket. Acute abscesses of such teeth easily form a sinus into the antrum following the course of least resistance. This condition, of course, has acute inflammation of the antrum as its sequel.

Sinus for Acute Alveolar Abscess to the Nasal Cavity. If an abscess on a superior incisor does not find relief by piercing the periosteum and gum, a sinus may be formed to the inferior meatus of the nose.

COMPLICA-TIONS *Acute Osteomyelitis,* or destruction of the cancellous part of the bone, occurs always during the formation of an acute apical alveolar abscess. The disease spreads easily in the spongiosa of the bone and the neighboring teeth are usually affected and are considerably loosened. If radical treatment is not undertaken at an early time, it may terminate in pyemia or septicemia, with fatal result.

Ostitis, or death of the bone, cell by cell, may be caused by prolonged subperiosteal parulis where the pus finds no escape and destroys the outer plate of the bone. After reaching the cancellous part of the bone it continues as osteomyelitis, which is not different from the osteomyelitis which starts from within.

Necrosis, or the death of bone *en masse,* is also frequently the result of the acute alveolar abscess. Necrosis may start from without by subperiosteal parulis where the blood supply from the periosteum is cut off by the pus which separates it from the bone. It may also start from within the bone by osteomyelitis, as a result of alveolar abscesses. It most always attacks the facial wall of the bone and is not often very extensive. The necrosed

PLATE VIII

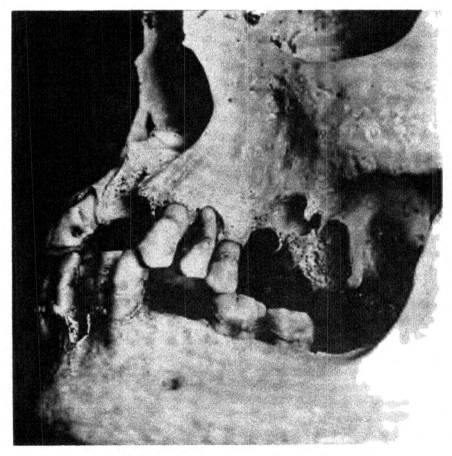

FIG. 32.—Skull showing large bone destruction due to abscesses.

F<small>IG</small>. 33

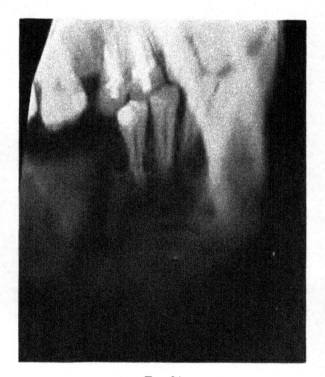

F<small>IG</small>. 34

F<small>IG</small>. 33.—Ostitis of the hard palate caused by a tooth.

F<small>IG</small>. 34.—Osteomyelitis of the mandible caused by an abscess on the lower first molar. The molar was extracted before the patient came under the author's observation.

part detaches from the healthy bone by absorption, the dead part being called a sequestrum. Pus discharges from a sequestrum in great amount until it is removed.

Resolution. Return to the normal will **TERMINATION** not occur without early therapeutic measures.

Scar Bone. Frequently we find conditions which have become chronic and in which a certain amount of repair has taken place, usually leaving but a comparatively small area of lessened density immediately around the apices of the roots. This new bone which fills in the area destroyed during the stage of active suppuration, is very much more dense than normal bone and appears in radiographs as a lighter area of denser structure. This is called scar bone. (Figure 37.)

Chronic Alveolar Abscess. After the pus has forced a sinus through the soft tissue, the swelling slowly subsides, and the flow of pus diminishes, the condition then passing into the chronic stage. Inflammatory granulation tissue is formed as an attempt of healing, which becomes enclosed by fibrous tissue to prevent the involving of larger areas.

Active Sinus. The suppuration, however, continues and the discharge flows through the original sinus or finds a new and shorter way, through the tissue which has been rendered more or less immune during the stage of acute inflammation. The walls of the sinus become fibrous forming an adhesion between the abscess cavity and the gum, or if the sinus leads to the face, between the abscess cavity and the skin. The skin on these places appears, therefore, fixed to the bone; it is drawn towards the diseased root apex in funnel fashion. This depression harbors the mouth of the sinus at its deepest point. Chronic abscesses discharge products of suppuration in large or small amount for months and years.

Closed Sinus. The mouth of the sinus of a chronic alveolar abscess sometimes becomes closed during a period of inhibition of pus formation. This is especially apt to occur if the discharge starts to drain through another

passage, such as is the case if an opening occurs into the
root canal when the process of decay breaks down the
tooth. This not only gives relief to the discharge from
the chronic abscess, but also relieves the primary source
of infection due to the death of the dental pulp. The
clinical picture of this condition is similar to the one of
the blind abscess, with the exception of a scar on the gum
or upon the face, formed by the closing of the mouth of
the sinus. This sort of chronic abscess without sinus is,
however, always a sequel to the acute abscess, while the
true blind abscess is formed in an entirely different way,
as we will see later.

Subacute Alveolar Abscesses. The closing of the sinus
by the process of granulation, during a period when suppuration is subdued or drained through a cavity via the
root canal, is usually not a stationary condition. The
cavity may become closed up by food debris, or the infection may become active again. This happens particularly during a period of lowered resistance, as during
pregnancy, when all the effort of the system is directed
to other parts. In recurring cases, this secondary process of suppuration is similar to the primary one. The
pus accumulates in the cancellous part of the bone, the
granulation tissue is destroyed, the sinus is reopened, or
a new outlet is formed to drain the discharge. The symptoms of the inflammation are, however, much less acute;
oedematic infiltration seldom occurs because the tissue
has been rendered more or less immune by previous attacks. A subacute attack usually quiets down after
a while and the condition continues as a chronic abscess
with sinus, or the sinus may even become closed again.
Such changes are liable to be repeated innumerable times
with irregular intervals of quietude.

Exostosis of the Root. The fibres of the periodontal
membrane have a great power of resistance and usually
they escape destruction if there is early and sufficient
drainage of the acute alveolar abscess. But if a chronic
periodontitis persists the cementoblasts are stimulated
by irritation from the chronic inflammation to deposit

PLATE X

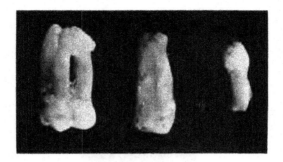

FIG. 35

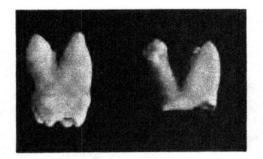

FIG. 36

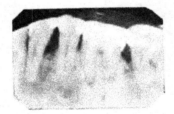

FIG. 37

FIGS. 35 and 36.—Photographs of teeth showing
exostosis of the root.

FIG. 37.—Molar with scar bone.

PLATE XI

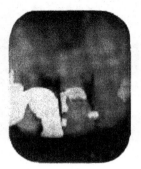

FIG. 38

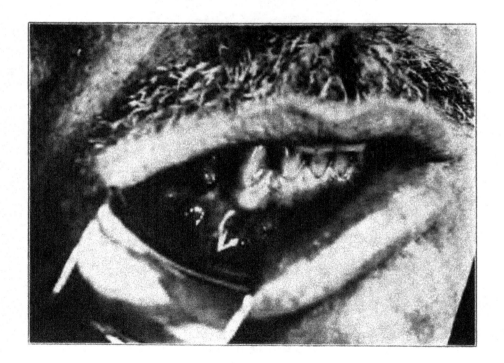

FIG. 39

FIG. 38.—Central incisor with acute abscess showing large bone destruction.
FIG. 39.—Photograph of sub-gingival parulis caused by first bicuspid.

new cementum causing hypercementosis, which is usually restricted to the place of disease, namely, the apex of the root. This thickening or bulging of the root is called exostosis and histologically shows an accumulation of lamellae of cementum containing an abundance of cement corpuscles and Haversian canals.

Necrosis of the Root. In cases where the parulis has been severe, and the formation of a sinus retarded, as is almost always the case in prolonged subperiosteal parulis, we usually get destruction of the apical part of the periodontal membrane. The cement of the tooth is then exposed and the denuded area shows a rough surface from contact with pus, and if the chronic alveolar abscess lasts a long time the root becomes discolored, having first a greenish, and later an almost black appearance. Absorption of tooth substance takes place at the apex which shows a ragged appearance if the tooth is extracted. The hard substances of the tooth have not the power to divide and expel diseased fragments, as in bone, but we will have to consider this absorption as a process of necrosis. The whole tooth represents the sequestrum, dead bone, cut off entirely from the blood supply which nourished it, from the inside through the pulp and from the outside through the periodontal membrane. In long standing chronic conditions, where the whole periodontal membrane has been destroyed, the tooth has the true appearance of dead tissue, the cementum of the whole root having a greenish black appearance.

DIAGNOSIS *Acute Periodontitis.* Local Symptoms: If the periodontal membrane becomes infected from a septic pulp, the tooth becomes very tender, the beating of the pulse can be felt by the patient, and the tooth protrudes out of the socket. The pain is felt principally at night. Cold and hot food have no influence, but mastication causes great pain because the tooth is, as the patient expresses it, too long.

Clinical signs: The tooth which causes the trouble is sensitive or even extremely painful on percussion; often it is also more or less loose.

Radiographic examination: The radiograph at this stage of the disease shows a dark shadow of the thickened periodontal membrane.

Acute Alveolar Abscess. Local symptoms: The stage of acute periodontitis is usually of very short duration. If relief does not come at once the pus will collect and form an acute abscess. The symptoms seem similar to the ones of acute periodontitis. Pain is very persistent and increases in severity; it is constant, deep and throbbing, sometimes excruciating. Hyperemia of the adjacent tissue sometimes is so marked as to loosen the neighboring teeth. Oedematic swelling of the neighboring parts occurs.

General symptoms: There is usually a marked rise in temperature; fever up to 104° F. is not uncommon. Chills may precede the fever and general malaise accompanies the disease.

Clinical signs: If an alveolar abscess has formed, the neighboring teeth usually become tender and it is difficult sometimes to find out which tooth has started the trouble. As the abscess starts from a diseased pulp, we can diagnose the case by testing the vitality of the pulp. A discolored tooth or a tooth with a large filling should be suspected. But to find out definitely we can apply the ice test; vital teeth give a reaction. The galvanic or the high frequency current can also be used. The teeth are dried and rendered isolated by putting a piece of celluloid or rubber-dam between their contact points; the galvanic current is then applied. If the galvanic current is used, one electrode is held in the hand and the other, surrounded by cotton saturated with normal salt solution, is applied first to a healthy tooth. The patient notes the sensation the current produces in the healthy tooth. The teeth that are suspected are then examined in the same manner and if a tooth gives no reaction it can be concluded that its pulp is diseased. If a high frequency apparatus is at hand, we let a small spark jump at the suspected tooth, dried and isolated in the manner just described. Pain caused signifies that the pulp is healthy, as a diseased pulp gives no such reaction.

Radiographic examination: Radiographs usually show distinct areas of lessened density where the bone has been destroyed by the process of suppuration. However, infiltration of the cancellous part of the bone is sometimes visible on account of the fluoroscopic properties of the pus. The apex of the diseased tooth usually occupies the centre of the area. In the upper jaw where the apices are close to the surface, so that the pus may easily find an outlet and accumulate under the periosteum and gum without destroying a large amount of bone, sometimes, even destroying no bone at all, we may find no area of lessened density at all, the bone appearing perfectly normal.

Alveolar Parulis. Local symptoms: After the pus has penetrated the bone, it accumulates under the periosteum, causing a flat swelling. In appearance the gum is highly inflamed and red, and the pain becomes very intense. Great relief usually occurs as soon as the pus penetrates the periosteum, when the high pressure is relieved and the pus collects under the gum, producing a ball-like swelling. If the abscess is on the palatal side, this part usually presents an enormous swelling, while parulis occurring on the buccal and labial sides, which usually is the case, is accompanied by an extensive infiltration of the surrounding tissue. The oedema sometimes partly or even entirely closes the eye if the trouble is in the upper jaw, while in the lower jaw, the floor of the mouth, lower part of the cheek and neck are principally infiltrated. The localization of this oedema is characteristic of the location of the diseased tooth. From a molar or bicuspid in the upper jaw where the upper part of the cheek is involved the corner of the mouth is drawn upwards, while the swelling from the lower parts draws the mouth downward. If an abscess occurs at the front teeth the respective lip is swollen and protruding. The submaxillary and submental glands for the front teeth are almost always enlarged. When the pus is about to come to the surface we note that a yellowish spot appears. This is called pointing of the abscess. The abscess, however, does not always point near the tooth that is the principal cause. The pus sometimes travels under the periosteum for quite a distance and may penetrate at a convenient point quite remote from the place where it leaves the bone. A sinus discharging from the mucous membrane of the mouth or skin is not always connected with and caused by an abscessed tooth. Impacted teeth, sequestra, diseased salivary or lacrimal glands sometimes cause sinuses, but it is not difficult to ascertain the cause.

Differential diagnosis: The lesions which may be mistaken for parulis are those of epulis, gumma and cyst. A true parulis resulting from a diseased pulp may also be mistaken for a parulis caused by an impacted, partially or entirely unerupted tooth, or by an abscess caused by pyorrhoea without involvement of the pulp. There is usually little difficulty in making the right diagnosis. Benign epulis is of slow development without any painful symptoms; sarcoma in the mouth is very modified, and the only malignant epulis we have to consider is carcinoma. Patients with carcinoma usually have a neglected mouth, and the bad condition of the teeth and the swelling of the glands, frequently gives the clinical picture of parulis. The generalizing character of the carcinoma and the anamnesis of the disease helps in diagnosis, and in a questionable case the histopathological picture of a piece excised for examination will decisively answer the question. Gummata are slow in growth; the history and manifestations at other parts as well as the Wasserman test will give the desired information. Cysts are of slow growth and show no symptoms of inflammation; an exploratory puncture gives escape to a clear, yellowish, odorless fluid. The diagnosis of parulis by impacted, unerupted teeth and pyorrhoea will be described in another place. That sinuses may also derive from glands, necrosed bone and impacted or unerupted teeth has already been mentioned, while oedema of the face also occurs from the salivary glands, if their ducts are obstructed or if infection involves them.

General symptoms: Parulis formation is almost always accompanied by general malaise; fever reaches its highest mark during the stage of subperiosteal parulis, and leucocytosis is very marked. The patient gets worn out from pain and loss of sleep, but as soon as the pus finds an outlet, the health improves rapidly.

Clinical signs: The same that has been said for acute alveolar abscess and acute periodontitis is true for parulis. In addition we feel by digital examination a fluctuation which is especially marked in subgingival parulis. Pressing upon the swelling increases the pain considerably. If the abscess points or if a sinus has already been formed, there is little difficulty in making a diagnosis.

Radiographic Examination: The radiograph usually shows the amount of bony destruction and is employed to find which tooth is the causative factor, but in certain cases no areas of decreased density are visible. This is especially the case when the apices of the teeth are close to the outer surface, as in the upper central incisors. In extreme cases where films canot be put into the mouth and in cases with sinuses leading to the face, large extraoral pictures should be taken, as the cause is often far removed from the mouth of the sinus.

Chronic Alveolar Abscess. Local symptoms: The patient who always remembers and presents a history of the acute process almost always complains of subacute attacks, where the gum swells up slightly and pus empties into the mouth, and there is usually a sense of pressure and soreness of touch and lameness of the tooth.

General symptoms: The submaxillary and submental lymph glands are usually slightly enlarged. Complications such as tonsilitis, pharyngitis, and gastric and intestinal infections may occur due to pus which is discharged into the mouth, but infectious arthritis, endocarditis, toxemia, and other diseases may also set in, and these can be considered as general symptoms calling our attention to the causative factor. These complications will be considered in a special chapter.

Clinical signs: A sinus is almost always found on the gum, or face; if it has closed, there is a visible scar. Whether or not we have a healed condition, the extent of the lesion can only be ascertained, if the sinus is closed, by radiographic examination.

Radiographic diagnosis: The radiograph reveals the chronic abscess by an area of lessened density, it also discloses if there is exostosis or necrosis of the root apex, which is an important factor in the determination of the method of treatment.

2. PROLIFERATING PERIODONTITIS AND ITS SEQUELS

In the last decades, teeth have been devitalized for several reasons without realizing the danger of such proceedings. Dentists knew only of the mechanical difficulties encountered in extirpating pulps and filling of root canals. The result of imperfect root-canal work was, however, not known until radiography was developed for dental use. When the so-called areas of lessened density were shown in radiographs at the apices of devitalized teeth, little attention was paid to them; they were considered a neglible quantity because the patient had no alarming symptoms of disturbance and often not even the slightest discomfort, and it was considered good dentistry to retain such teeth rather than lose an important organ of mastication. But since the pathology and bacteriology of these symptomless lesions has been studied more carefully and since the important discovery of focal infection, we have come to realize the grave fact that such septic conditions about the teeth may be more dangerous than the violent acute conditions, principally on account of the fact that their deceiving nature undermines the patient's general health and causes, if conditions are right, secondary infections in other parts of the body, the nature of which we shall study in a special chapter.

DEFINITION *Proliferating periodontitis and its sequel, the granuloma,* are changes in which new formation of tissue from the periodontal membrane is the important feature; suppuration plays a secondary rôle

PLATE XII

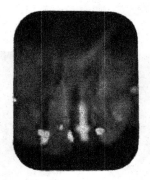

Fɪɢ. 40

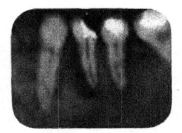

Fɪɢ. 41

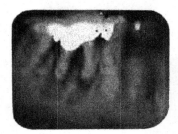

Fɪɢ. 42

Fɪɢ. 40.—Lateral granuloma.
Fɪɢ. 41.—Apical granuloma.
Fɪɢ. 42.—Interradial granuloma.

PLATE XIII

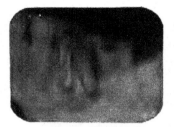

FIG. 43

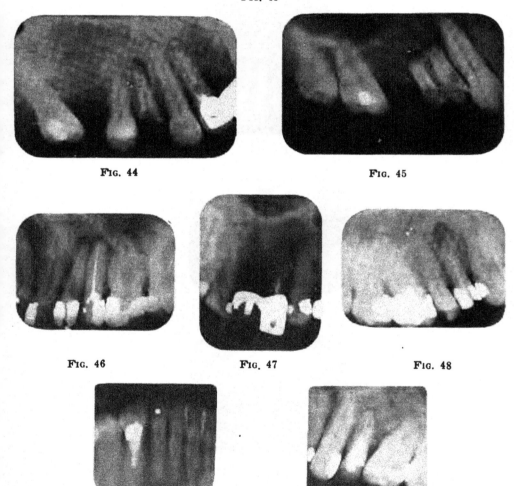

FIG. 44   FIG. 45

FIG. 46   FIG. 47   FIG. 48

FIG. 49   FIG. 50

FIGS. 43, 44 and 45.—Granulomata caused by decay of the tooth. There is free communication from the root canal into the mouth.

FIGS. 46, 47 and 48.—Granulomata caused by incomplete pulp extirpation.

FIGS. 49 and 50.—Granulomata due to broken instruments left in root canal.

and does not involve the surrounding tissues. It is characteristic that the condition starts without the patient's knowledge and without symptoms of inflammation.

VARIETIES *Apical Granuloma.* The most common seat of chronic periodontitis and its sequel and is the periapical region, at the outlet of the root canal from which the disease starts.

Lateral Granuloma. Sometimes teeth have accessory foramina as high as the middle of the root. These may become a source of trouble if the root canal has to be treated. Perforations by root canal instruments at the side of a root are, however, more frequently the cause of lateral abscesses.

Interradial Granuloma. The floor of the pulp chamber is sometimes penetrated in multirooted teeth by burrs or root-canal instruments, seldom by decay, causing granulomata or chronic abscesses between the roots. It it almost impossible to treat these interradial abscesses on account of anatomical difficulties.

ETIOLOGY Proliferating periodontitis is primarily caused as a protective reaction of the tissue against irritating excretions from the root canal, such as pus bacteria and toxins, or against injudicious application of irritating drugs, such as formaldehyde, sulphuric acid and other medicaments used during root canal treatment. Ulrich believes that haematogenous infection is the explanation for all apical abscesses with the probable exception of teeth which have been capped following caries. I fully believe that haematogenous infection is the cause in certain cases, especially those of infection or reinfection after medicinal treatment, leaving an area of lowered resistance in the periapical region, such as a periodontal membrane or a denuded or necrosed apex; but it seems to me very improbable that all or even a large amount of the cases should be due to this cause. The histopathological picture speaks so plainly for an irritating and infective source from the root canal, the fact that I discovered blind abscesses in persons in whom no other foci could be found after careful search, and the fact that the streptococcus, which is almost always found in the dentinal tubules, is also the bacteria which most frequently inhabits the granuloma, seem to me simpler and more probable reasons, especially where we have such an obvious source as the root canal from which infection may be continued.

The microörganisms which sooner or later invade the granuloma are never very large in number. Their virulence has usually been decreased by unfavorable conditions, such as lack of oxygen and lack of nutrition where most of the organic matter has been removed, and the blood supply is cut off. The result is a symptomless or chronic inflammation walled off by the fibrous sack enclosing the granuloma, containing lymphocytes and leucocytes.

Proliferating periodontitis can be caused whether the pulp chamber is open or closed and results from the following conditions:

Decay of the Tooth. If caries has destroyed the enamel and dentin, so that there is an opening into the pulp chamber, the products of decomposition have a chance to escape into the mouth. This prevents them from penetrating through the apical foramen thereby infecting the deeper tissues surrounding the root of the tooth. While the disease of the pulp progresses slowly towards the apex, protective measures are taken by the surrounding tissue against the poisonous substances of fermentation and decomposition. The periodontal membrane proliferates and forms a granuloma, and harbors in its center fluids of decomposition and absorption.

Incomplete Pulp Extirpation. The extirpation of the dental pulp is an operation which should not be undertaken except after serious consideration of its necessity and most careful prognostic study of the case. Our present knowledge of the alveolar abscess should warn us of the possible consequences of such an operation and teach us to make the greatest effort to save the pulp by prophylactic as well as by therapeutic means. A tooth should be radiographed to diagnose if a root is straight or bent and to ascertain the size, length, direction, and branching of the root canals. Some teeth are bent to such an extent, or their root canals are so obstructed by secondary deposits of dentin or pulp stones, that we are not able to remove the pulp entirely, no matter how skilled the operator and how much time is spent. We stand therefore before an impossible task. Among these cases belong many teeth which have moved forward during childhood on account of loss of an anterior tooth and these teeth have been moved for large distances for orthodontic purposes. This may result in bent roots. Most of the permanent teeth erupt long before the calcification of their roots is finished, and if force is applied at the stage of root formation, it will move the calcified part and bend the uncalcified apical region.

If parts of diseased pulp are left to remain in the roots, in branches of the root canal, apical part or accessory foramina, this organic matter will, after the tooth has been filled, stimulate proliferation of the periodontal membrane and cause a granuloma. If a healthy tooth has to be devitalized to give attachment to bridge work or to remove pulp stones which cause neuralgia, the remaining pulp particles are often infected by careless treatment, or by bacteria supplied by the blood stream. The condition then is the same as if the pulp had been infected in the first place.

Inefficient Root-canal Treatment. Root canals which have not been sufficiently treated previous to the insertion of the root filling, are liable to cause the same result as just described. After all the organic matter has been removed by mechanical and chemical means, we must still consider the bacteria which are growing in the microscopic dentinal tubules and the accessory apical foramina. These should be destroyed by antiseptics [ionic treatment with iodine was found specially helpful by the writer] or they will become the source of infection, which is especially favored by incomplete or poorly condensed root canal fillings. The same condition occurs if root canal

instruments are broken and left in the canals. They ob-
struct the way to the apical part which is left in a septic
and unfilled condition.

Inefficient Root-canal Fillings. A root-canal filling
which is perfect should seal the apical foramen hermetically so that no infection can pass from the tooth into the
surrounding tissues. Scrupulous asepsis is also of greatest importance, not only during root-canal treatment, but
also during root-canal filling. If the filling leaves a space
at the apex containing organic matter, moisture, or air,
or if the filling material is of such a nature that it shrinks,
irritates or relies on antiseptic properties, which wear
out with time, it gives chance for bacterial growth.

Invasion of Bacteria. It may also be caused by invasion of bacteria, reaching the pulp by way of the dentinal
tubules, which can be easily entered if the enamel has
been removed. If this is the case several factors must
be reckoned with. Danger of infection is certain if the
tooth is young and if it must be greatly reduced to fit a
crown, because the dentinal tubules in this case are larger,
less calcified, and nearer the pulp. If these little wounds
(sections through the dentinal tubules) are not carefully
protected during the preparation of the tooth and during
the time which elapses until the crown is set, bacteria
which abound in the mouth will invade these dentinal
tubules, multiply, and progress even after the crown has
been set, until they reach the pulp and cause suppurative
pulpitis.

Death of Pulp without Access of Air. It is a well-
known fact that the pulp of a tooth may become diseased
because the irritating action of certain fillings forms
progressive decay under a filling or a gold or porcelain
jacket crown. It is usually due to lack of oxygen that
such cases proceed in a chronic manner and often large
apical granulomata are formed without symptoms of
disease. If the pulp of such teeth is opened, it often
results in a violent subacute attack due to the change in
the oxygen tension.

PLATE XIV

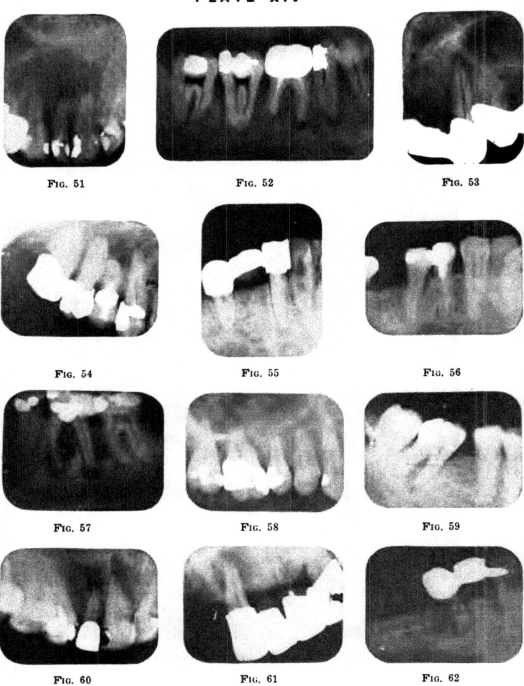

FIG. 51 FIG. 52 FIG. 53

FIG. 54 FIG. 55 FIG. 56

FIG. 57 FIG. 58 FIG. 59

FIG. 60 FIG. 61 FIG. 62

FIGS. 51, 52, 53, 54, 55 and 56.—Granulomata caused by inefficient root canal fillings.
FIGS. 57, 58 and 59.—Granulomata from decay under fillings without access of air.
FIGS. 60, 61 and 62.—Granulomata occurring on crowned teeth.

PLATE XV

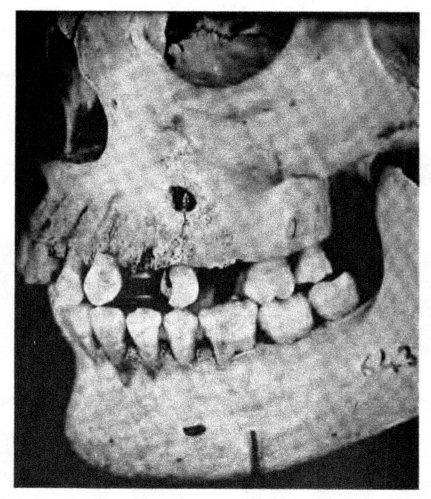

Fig. 63.—Skull of Italian showing bony destruction caused by an apical granuloma on the left upper second bicuspid.

Haematogenous Infection. Granulomata usually are due to direct entrance of the disease through the root canal but may also be caused as a secondary manifestation due to bacteremia, that is, the presence of the microörganisms in the blood. Any devitalized tooth has around its apex a place of lowered resistance with lowered oxygen tension due to the destruction of nerve and blood supply of the apex and contiguous bone areas, a destruction which may have been caused by the use of caustic and irritating drugs for root canal medication or the destructive process of suppuration.

COURSE OF THE DISEASE *Proliferating Periodontitis.* The poisonous products of bacterial decomposition and fermentation reach the peripheral tissues of the tooth and stimulate protective new growth. If the tooth is extracted at this stage we find a marked thickening of slightly reddish character at the apical region.

Granuloma. The proliferation usually goes on until the new growth has reached the size of a pea. Larger granulomata are, however, not uncommon; they may reach the size of a robin's egg. A fibrous layer surrounds the lesion, which is very thick in the beginning and firmly attached to the healthy part of the periodontal membrane. The extracted tooth usually carries with it such a granuloma, or so-called abscess sack. Later, when the granuloma reaches larger sizes, it becomes thinner and is often destroyed by fatty degeneration, which decreases its resisting power to suppuration. In the center we find the seat of chronic inflammation, harboring often a small amount of pus or other products of degeneration and absorption, which are usually taken up by the lymph or capillary system. Destruction of bone depends upon the progress of the chronic inflammation. In the upper jaw, where the apices of the roots are close to the facial surface of the bone, the alveolar plate is almost always destroyed; in the lower jaw it is a most infrequent occurrence to find the thick cortical layers of the mandible involved. If the tooth is extracted at this stage the abscess will usually remain in the jaw and has to be removed by careful curettage.

The microörganisms which inhabit the granuloma have to struggle for their existence in this tissue which is formed by lymphocytes, leucocytes, and fibroblasts; pus, therefore, is formed only in very minute quantity.

Subacute Attacks. At one time or another the suppuration may become more active and destroy the fibrous tissue of the granuloma. The causes of such acute bacterial activity may be lowered resistance of the body and wearing out of the cells, whose function is to destroy foreign bodies. It may come from a change in oxygen tension, a thing with which almost every dentist is familiar, namely, an acute attack after opening into the pulp chamber of the tooth which gives the air a chance to enter. It also may be caused by haematogenous infection, the invasion of another kind of bacteria, causing a mixed infection. In these subacute attacks the pus usually burrows a sinus to the gum, the tissues react, not, however, very actively, as in the acute abscess, because partial immunization has taken place in the tissues surrounding the chronic condition. After the pus has evacuated, the signs of inflammation usually disappear without treatment and the sinus closes up. This, however, does not indicate that the abscess has now completely healed, but only signifies that pus formation has decreased and granulation predominates, which may be reversed at any favorable time.

Exostosis of the Root. If the fibers of the granuloma persist for a long time, so that the metabolism of the cementum is not interfered with, the constant irritation from the chronic inflammation stimulates the activity of the cementoblasts which results in new formation of cementum, which we call exostosis of the root. This usually results in a bulbous form at the apex which makes extraction extremely difficult.

Necrosis of the Root. If the apical part of the periodontal membrane has been destroyed, the nutrient

PLATE XVI

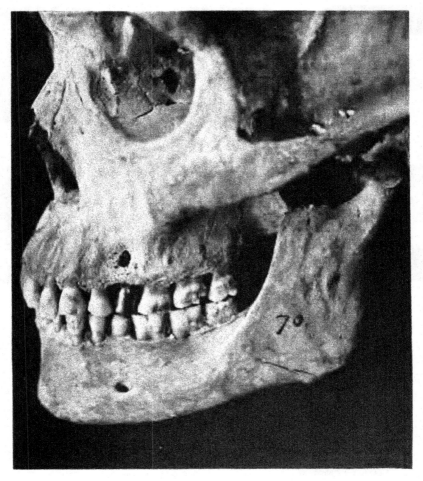

FIG. 64.—Skull showing bony destruction due to a granuloma caused by a left upper bicuspid, bearing a gold crown.

PLATE XVII

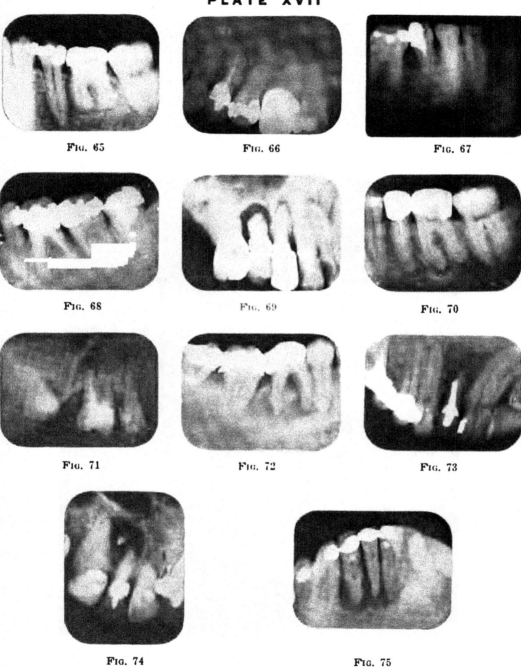

FIG. 65   FIG. 66   FIG. 67

FIG. 68   FIG. 69   FIG. 70

FIG. 71   FIG. 72   FIG. 73

FIG. 74   FIG. 75

FIGS. 65, 66, 67, 68, 69 and 70.—Radiographs of teeth with granulomata showing marked exostosis of the roots.

FIGS. 71, 72 and 73.—Radiographs of teeth with necrosed apices due to granulomata.

FIGS. 74 and 75.—Radiographs of teeth showing large osteomyelitic area.

supply of the tooth is doubly cut off. The cementum, which at this stage contains numerous accessory apical foramina and Haversian canals, soon becomes infected and necrosed. The condition then is that of bone with the periosteum raised and no blood supply from within. Here such areas become separated and are expelled as sequestra. In the tooth this cannot take place, and we must consider the whole organ as the sequestrum which is retained by the remaining periodontal membrane at the cervical part of the root. In some cases, chronic inflammation of the remaining periodontal membrane sets in, causing necrosis of the entire root, which then has a greenish appearance, a condition which is often spoken of as "gangrene of the root."

TERMINA-TION *Resolution.* The condition of chronic abscess may be considered the termination for the larger percentage of the cases; it may continue for years. Resolution never occurs without treatment.

Chronic Osteomyelitis. The bone destruction, occurring as a result of the inflammatory granulation, involves an osteomyelitis even at its early stages. Fortunately, nature in most cases prevents an extensive involvement by circumscribing the lesion with a protective layer of fibrous tissue enclosing the seat of inflammation, as will be shown later in microscopic pictures. Osteomyelitis produced by such conditions is much less severe than in other parts of the body and frequently symptomless.

Cysts. There has been much writing by German scientists tracing root cysts of larger or smaller dimensions back to epitheliated granulomata. Dependorf* has devoted a large amount of time to the study of the development of such cysts. He says that not all epitheliated granulomata will become cysts, and that cyst formation depends on a partial and concentric degeneration of the inner part of the granuloma first of all; secondly, dependent on epithelium which is able to develop and proliferate, and thirdly, due to the interference with the blood supply, due

* *See* Bibliography.

to the chronic inflammatory conditions. The growth of the cyst is dependent upon chronic inflammatory conditions, which are enclosed in the lumen and which cause degeneration of the larger or smaller parts of the central core. The inner surface becomes lined with epithelium and the cyst may develop to almost any dimension. It is the author's opinion that cysts may form from epitheliated granulomata, although judging from the number of granulomata which do not form cysts, we may draw the conclusion that such a formation is decidedly rare.

DIAGNOSIS *Proliferating Periodontitis.* Local symptoms: It is characteristic of the proliferating periodontitis that it occurs and grows without causing any local symptoms. The tooth is not elongated because the growth occurs at the expense of the bone. Sometimes, however, the patient has a sense of pressure over the tooth and often the pulsation of the blood is felt in the vascular granulation tissue around the apex, especially after violent exercise.

General symptoms: In the beginning stage there is rarely any systemic involvement, although the writer has procured streptococci cultures from many apices of teeth which in radiographs showed only the slightest indication of proliferating periodontitis. In a hospital case of endocarditis such a small area prevented entire recovery and the removal was followed by rapid improvement.

Clinical signs: There are no signs which would indicate proliferating periodontitis.

Radiographic examination: With the intraoral radiograph we can diagnose the early stages of periodontitis. The dark line around the contour of the root which represents the periodontal membrane is thickened at the apex, and in later stages we find distinct areas of lessened density which indicate loss of bone taken up by the proliferation of the periodontal membrane.

Granuloma. Local symptoms: The granuloma very frequently gives no symptoms; a sense of pressure and lameness of the tooth may be noticed occasionally.

General symptoms: At this stage we frequently find complications due to the absorption of toxins and bacteria. Malaise, a tired feeling, and inability to do a day's work is a frequent indication of an intoxication which may come from oral lesions besides all the other complications mentioned in the previous chapter. These conditions should be recognized and inquired into and looked at as a reason for careful diagnosis of the mouth by means of radiographs.

Clinical signs: As clinical signs are absent at this stage, it is of greatest importance to rely on radiographic diagnosis.

Radiographic examination: The granuloma shows in the radiograph as a circumscribed area of decreased density and is easily recognized when present at the apex of a devitalized tooth. While there is usually little doubt about the location of an abscess on a single-rooted tooth, it is often more difficult to make a correct diagnosis on multirooted teeth, especially the upper ones. The upper first bicuspids should be radiographed from a buccomesial direction, while two radiographs are necessary to show distinctly the condition of the two buccal roots and the palatal root. The first is taken about perpendicular to the buccal roots, the other perpendicular to the palatal root.

Subacute Attacks. Local symptoms: If suppuration becomes more active in the granuloma, the patient often feels a grumbling and lameness of the tooth which may disappear after several days. In other instances, the wall of the granuloma is broken down, resulting in a regular subacute attack. The patient then experiences the symptoms of the acute abscess, pain, redness, fever, and swelling. The tissue, however, has been rendered more or less immune, and the symptoms of inflammation are more modified, sometimes hardly noticeable, at other times extreme. The condition, however, will usually pass through the stages of parulis until a sinus occurs on the gum to give exit to the accumulating pus.

General symptoms: The general symptoms depend upon how severe and acute the attack is. There may be none at all, or they may be equal to an acute process passing through the stages of parulis.

Clinical signs: When the gum over the abscess is found to be swollen and in subacute condition, the guilty tooth is usually easily located. When the pulp has been dead for a long time, electric tests will give negative results, while in acute conditions there is usually some doubt, especially if the nerve fibres of the pulp have not been entirely destroyed. The patient usually tells upon questioning a history of previous attacks or treatment of the tooth.

Radiographic examination: Radiographs will reveal an area of lessened density on a devitalized and partly filled root. This is the important feature of differentiation between an acute attack, where the pulp has been diseased only recently and where there is no evidence of previous root-canal work.

PLATE XVIII

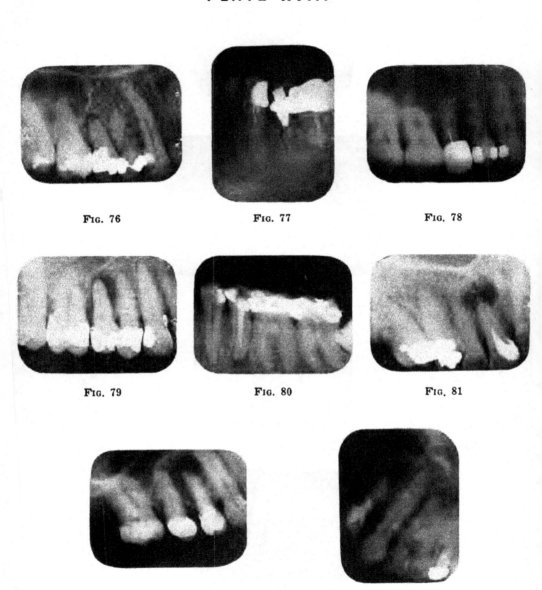

FIG. 76   FIG. 77   FIG. 78

FIG. 79   FIG. 80   FIG. 81

FIG. 82   FIG. 83

FIGS. 76 and 77.—Radiographs of teeth showing small areas of lessened density indicating periodontitis.

FIGS. 79, 80 and 81.—Radiographs of teeth showing large areas of lessened density indicating granulomata.

FIGS. 82 and 83.—Radiographs of teeth with subacute abscesses. The root canals of the teeth have been partly filled, indicating chronic disease of long standing.

PLATE XIX

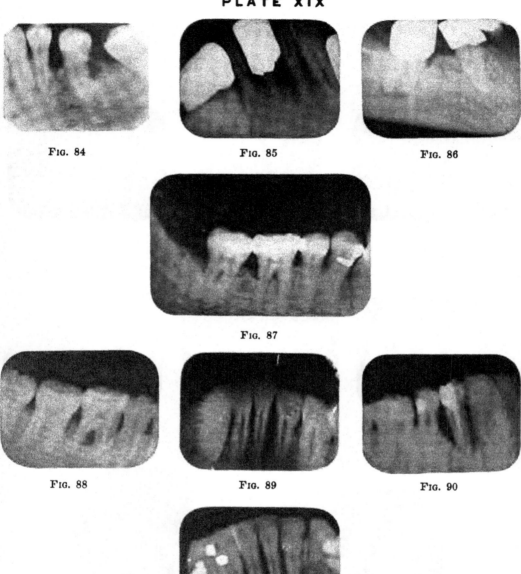

FIG. 84   FIG. 85   FIG. 86

FIG. 87

FIG. 88   FIG. 89   FIG. 90

FIG. 91

FIGS. 84, 85 and 86.—Radiographs of teeth showing dark areas about their necks representing pus pockets caused by mechanical injury.

FIGS. 87, 88, 89 and 90.—Radiographs of teeth showing dark areas indicating pus pockets at the alveolar border.

FIG. 91.—Radiograph showing a lower incisor with an apical abscess caused by pus pockets, mesial as well as distal. The tooth is vital.

CHAPTER IV

PATHOLOGICAL DEVELOPMENT AND DIAGNOSIS OF ALVEOLAR ABSCESSES DUE TO OTHER CAUSES THAN THE DISEASE OF THE DENTAL PULP

We have noted in the preceding chapter that the largest percentage of the oral abscesses are due to diseases of the dental pulp. However, other forms of abscesses in and around the alveolar process occur which are due to different causes. These sometimes give almost the same symptoms as some of the already described types and it is important to distinguish them because their treatment is so widely different.

According to the etiological factor we can distinguish alveolar abscesses due to diseases of the gum and alveolar abscesses due to difficult eruption, impaction and unerupted teeth.

1. *Alveolar Abscesses due to Diseases of the Gum.*

ETIOLOGY *Injury of the Gum.* The gum is occasionally injured by the use of a toothpick or a bristle of a toothbrush which may become lodged between the gingival margin and the tooth. An inflammation may occur if the wound had been infected, involving not only the gum but frequently the cervical part of the periodontal membrane and the periosteum, resulting in a marginal periodonditis with subgingival parulis formation. Other causes are poor fillings, either projecting into the gum or lacking in contour, faulty bands and gold crowns, which project into the gum instead of being closely fitted around the neck of the tooth. After the cement by which they are fastened has washed away, these places will harbor contaminated food and be the seat of fermentation and later suppuration. A similar condition occurs under fixed bridges, which can be properly cleaned neither by patient nor dentist, the gum becomes inflamed, and after the removal of the bridge we often discover an extensive ulcerated area. The vile odor which is released after removing such appliances speaks for itself and makes superfluous further comment as to its unsanitary and disease breeding properties.

Pus Pockets. Pus pockets such as are characteristic of pyorrhoea alveolaris sometimes become closed up. This, or any other reason which prevents the pus from escaping at the cervical margin, causes accumulation of pus or abscess formation.

COURSE OF THE DISEASE In abscesses caused by injury of the gum, the infection is usually superficial. The pus is seldom formed under the periosteum, but accumulates between the periosteum and gum in the submucosa of the mucous membrane. A red swelling is formed at the gingival margin, a small parulis, which heals spontaneously after it breaks or after an incision is made. In more deep-seated cases the ligamentum circulare and periodontal membrane may become infiltrated. The Haversian canals then become infected, causing destruction of the cervical part of the alveolar process. If pus pockets such as occur in pyorrhoea alveolaris or other forms of marginal periodontitis are the cause of the abscess, the accumulation of pus is usually more deeply seated than in the case of injury of the gum. On account of the closure of the natural outlet at the cervical margin the pus will invade the alveolar process and find its way to the surface of the gum. The process usually passes through the stages of subperiosteal and subgingival parulis, which, however, gives no very severe symptoms as the tissues have been pretty well immunized by the long existing chronic inflammation. This destructive process may, however, be halted any time if the outlet at the gum margin is reopened, when the disease continues in its former chronic form.

DIAGNOSIS Local and general symptoms: The patient experiences about the same discomfort as in the parulis formation already described, only perhaps in a modified way, because the tissue has almost always been more or less immunized by a preëxisting and causative chronic condition, as in pyorrhoea, or because the abscess is very superficial and little destruction is necessary to form an outlet for the discharge.

Clinical signs: Upon examination, a tumor-like swelling is seen nearer the gum margin than in true alveolar abscess and parulis. The surrounding tissues are less involved. There is usually no history of pulp disease; the tooth may be vital or devitalized. The patient often remembers that the gum had been injured or there may be indication of pyorrhoea from the general condition of the mouth. The differential diagnosis may be established by the radiograph.

Radiographic examination: Very often we are left in doubt, whether we have to deal with a true alveolar abscess, caused by a diseased pulp, or whether the condition is wholly periodontal. Especially doubtful cases are those where the tooth has a gold crown or large fillings, as both are conditions which indicate the involvement of the pulp. The importance of knowing whether the pulp is involved or not is evident if we consider the first and most important therapeutic measure, the removal of the cause. A radiograph will help a great deal in diagnosis; if there is no area of lessened density at the apex of the tooth, we know that the abscess is not formed from a dead pulp, and often we see a large dark area at the neck of the tooth indicating marginal destruction of the alveolar process due to a gingival abscess or parulis.

2. *Alveolar Abscess Due to Difficult Eruption, Impaction or Unerupted Teeth.*

ETIOLOGY *Difficult eruption and partial impaction:* The lower third molar is the tooth which most frequently is impacted, but also the upper third molar is often in irregular position. The reason is that the

third molars are the last teeth to take their places in the
dental area, and as the jaw is often too short (a result of
civilization) to accommodate all the teeth, the third molar
becomes locked under the bulging of the crown of the
second molar.   In the lower jaw there is an additional-.
obstacle, the ascending ramus, the terminal boundary of
the part of the mandible that accommodates the teeth.
The cuspid teeth are the next in the series which are most
likely to be impacted, the reason being that the tooth in
abnormal conditions does not appear until long after the
lateral incisors and the first bicuspids are in place.   While
the lower third molars and cuspids are most likely to be
impacted, any tooth in the lower as well as the upper jaw
may become impacted if the space which they are to oc-
cupy is taken up by other teeth, or if the malposition has
been assumed at an early period during the development
of the tooth germ.

Inflammation may start before the tooth has pierced
the gum, from the irritation caused by biting on the tissue
overlying the occlusal surface of the tooth.   In most
cases, however, the infection occurs after the gum has
been pierced by the erupting cusps and may be due to
food and fluids of the mouth entering through this wound.
The soft tissue does not adhere to the enamel of the crown,
as it does to the cementum on the root by means of the
periodontal membrane and ligamentum circulare, and
therefore foreign material is free to pass deep into the
tissue around, slowly erupting teeth both impacted and
normal.   In other cases the infection is due more to irritation of the gum, which is crowded over the occlusal surface during mastication and becomes bruised by the teeth
of the opposite jaw.   In such conditions inflammation
again sets in and is maintained.

Unerupted Impacted Teeth.   In some cases teeth grow
in an entirely horizontal or even downward direction
and are so interlocked, that it is impossible for them to
come to the surface.   Such teeth may lie dormant for
several years but at any time may suddenly become associated with active pathological conditions, when exert-
ing pressure on the tissue towards which they grow.   It

PLATE XX

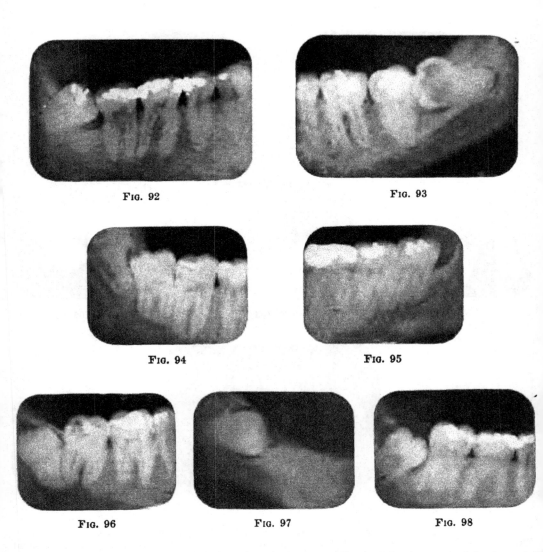

FIG. 92

FIG. 93

FIG. 94

FIG. 95

FIG. 96

FIG. 97

FIG. 98

FIGS. 92, 93, 94 and 95.—Radiograph showing dark areas indicating abscesses caused by impacted but partly erupted wisdom teeth. In Fig. 93 the pulp has been involved and periodontitis caused at the apex.

FIG. 96, 97 and 98.—Radiographs of unerupted molars showing dark areas indicating abscesses.

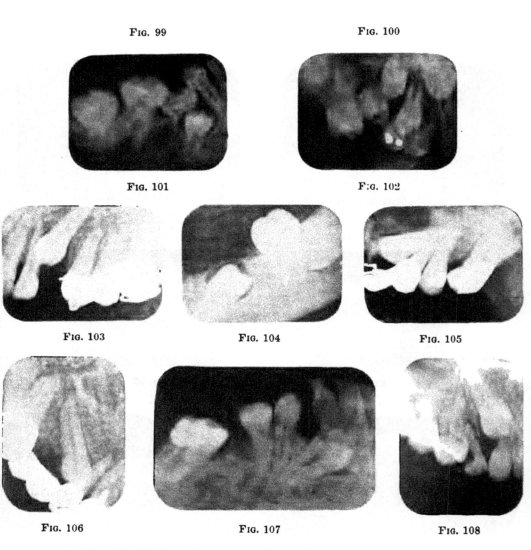

Fig. 99

Fig. 100

Fig. 101

F:g. 102

Fig. 103

Fig. 104

Fig. 105

Fig. 106

Fig. 107

Fig. 108

FIG. 99.—Radiograph showing impacted second and third molar.
FIG. 100.—Radiograph shows impacted second molar which had been broken off. The third molar is partly erupted and prevents the second molar from coming up.
FIGS. 101 and 102.—Radiographs show impacted temporary molars.
FIGS. 103, 104, 105, 106, 107 and 108.—Radiographs show other impactions causing more or less troub

seems to be a physio-pathological law that any abnormal pressure in the body causes resorption of the part most easily dissolved. This in turn forms a place of lowered resistance and is liable to infection. Infection may occur from a blind abscess on a neighboring tooth or through the blood.

COURSE OF THE DISEASE After the infection has taken place the process of inflammation may take on a chronic course. This is especially the case if there is an outlet for the pus through the gingival opening made by the erupting tooth. This outlet, however, is rarely adequate, pus is accumulated and when under pressure is forced deeper into the bone as well as into the soft tissue. The inflammation then extends to the adjoining parts, involving the fauces, mucous membrane and muscles about the ramus. A pharyngitis often sets in, trismus of the muscles of mastication is of common occurrence, and deglutition becomes difficult. The abscess usually passes through the stages of alveolar parulis, and the trismus becomes so marked that the patient is unable to open his mouth. At this time usually there is a sinus formed, the pus evacuates and the movements of the jaw become less constrained. If no surgical procedure restores the condition to normal, the patient may have recurrent attacks of the same character at frequent intervals. If the impacted tooth causes absorption of another tooth, this is sometimes carried so far as to involve its pulp. Such conditions cause severe neuralgic pains, and if the pulp becomes infected severe alveolar abscesses.

DIAGNOSIS Local symptoms: The local symptoms are usually well marked but not characteristic or distinctive of the cause. There is intense pain, sometimes almost unbearable, referred to the ear, eye, forehead, or opposite jaw. If the condition is due to a third molar, the patient complains of a sore throat and inability to swallow; often the mouth can be opened but very little. There may be extreme swelling of the face on the affected side; at other times the external swelling is less marked, all the infiltration being on the inside of the mouth.

General symptoms: There is usually fever up to 104°
F., general malaise, and the patient often presents serious
symptoms, especially if severe pain has caused continual
loss of sleep.

Clinical signs: If a third molar is the cause of the
trouble, examination of the mouth is often very difficult.
Ankylosis should be excluded, which is a disease of the
mandibular joints and is usually not accompanied by
severe pain or temperature.   Pus can frequently be
pressed from the swelling and often a white cusp is seen
sticking out from the inflamed gum. If we have to do
with an unerupted tooth the radiograph will be the only
means by which a positive diagnosis can be made.

Radiographic diagnosis: The radiograph is a most
valuable means of detecting the real cause of the trouble
and is furthermore a valuable aid in determining the
mode of operation. Partly erupted impacted teeth can
be taken on small, intraoral films, but unerupted teeth
should be taken on large extraoral films or plates, because
there is a possibility of malposition. Third molars have
been found in the ramus as far up as the mandibular notch
and as low down as the angle of the ramus, places which
cannot be reached with intraoral pictures. For impacted
upper teeth in the anterior region of the mouth, a large
film placed between the teeth with an exposure from well
above the head will give in most cases good results. For
impacted cuspids in the lower jaw the rays should be
directed somewhat from underneath, as these teeth are
often situated as low as the lower border of the mandible.
Stereoscopic radiographs would be more desirable in
many cases, as an ordinary radiograph is flat and does not
give the exact location of the tooth. For example, you
cannot tell whether the impacted cuspid in Figure 107 is
external or internal to the other teeth; however, the taking of stereo-radiographs requires a great deal of skill and
necessitates the use of special apparatus.   The stereo-
radiographic technique is still in the process of development; good results, however, can be obtained, and in difficult cases these pictures, which give a perspective view,
are of great value.

PLATE XXII

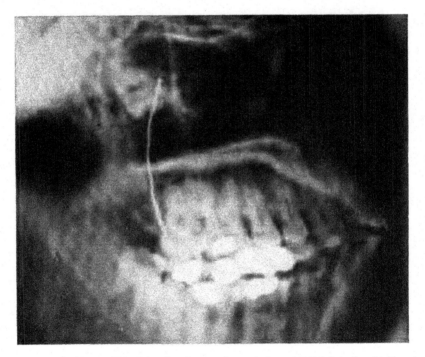

FIG. 109.—Radiographic plate showing an impacted upper third molar in the posterior wall of the antrum. Symptoms covering a period of one year prior to its discovery: Periodical unilateral headaches, with entire absence of pain, but bad taste in the mouth every morning. There is a sinus opening just back of the second molar. The tooth discharges half a dram of pus in twenty-four hours.

Reproduced by courtesy of Dr. Gibbons. Radiograph by Dr. A. W. George.

PLATE XXIII

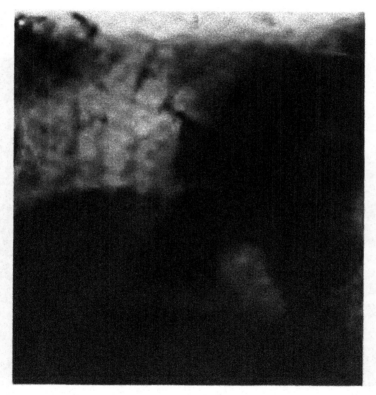

FIG. 110.—Radiographic plate by which an unerupted lower third molar was discovered at the angle of the jaw. Note the large cyst.

CHAPTER V

PATHOLOGICAL DEVELOPMENT AND DIAGNOSIS OF ABSCESSES OF THE TONGUE AND SALIVARY GLANDS AND DUCTS

Thus far abscesses occurring in and about the mandibular and maxillary bones have been described; these are by far the most common ones. The tongue and salivary glands are, however, occasionally the seat of abscess conditions.

1. ABSCESSES OF THE TONGUE

The tongue is comparatively rare as the seat of inflammation and infection, but if abscesses of the tongue occur, we have a condition which may bear grave results. Diffuse infiltration frequently occurs and often spreads to the posterior part of the tongue, and, on account of its increased size, causing difficulty in breathing which often can be relieved only by tracheotomy.

VARIETIES Three varieties of tongue abscesses shall be described.
1. The simple abscess of the tongue.
2. The phlegmonous abscess of the tongue.
3. The tubercular abscess of the tongue.

1. *The Simple Abscess of the Tongue.*

ETIOLOGY Circumscribed abscess formation of the tongue is very often due to injury or entrance into the tongue of a foreign body, such as a fish bone, during mastication. More often, however, there are sharp, broken-down teeth which cause the primary injury, and if such teeth are abscessed, discharging pus from sinus or pocket, the wound at once becomes infected.

CLINICAL COURSE The infection usually assumes a more or less chronic appearance, causing a tumor-like thickening at the infected part. If no therapeutic interference occurs, the abscess may break, but more frequently it will end in the phlegmonous type.

DIAGNOSIS Local symptoms: The simple abscess of the tongue causes more or less local discomfort. The place where the lesion occurs is extremely tender to touch, causing difficulty in eating and speaking.

Clinical signs: If the tongue is palpitated, one can feel distinctly a hard swelling in the substance of the lingual muscle; the tongue is usually slightly enlarged, which causes indentations on its sides because it is crowded into the interdental spaces. In the first stages it may be hard to differentiate this lesion from gummata and tumors, but later when the signs of inflammation are more marked and when there is discharge of pus, there is usually no doubt about the diagnosis. An exploratory incision or puncture may be made; this should be deep enough to reach the seat of trouble and will, if pus is drawn, verify the diagnosis.

2. *The Phlegmonous Abscess of the Tongue.*

ETIOLOGY Injuries due to infected foreign bodies, as already described, and injury from carious teeth surrounded by septic conditions very often take on a more acute form than the one just described. Progressive alveolar abscesses may also cause phlegmonous abscesses of the tongue, if their course involves the deeper, posterior lingual muscles.

In the phlegmonous abscess of the tongue, a purulent or fibrino-purulent infiltration, causes a diffuse swelling. The size of the tongue increases rapidly, the anterior part is pushed forward and no longer has room between the teeth. The soft palate and the mould are pushed

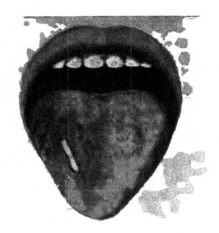

FIG. 111

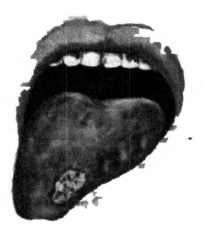

FIG. 112

FIG. 111.—Simple abscess of the tongue.
FIG. 112.—Tubercular abscess of the tongue.

upward and the epiglottis downward into the larynx. In severe cases, swallowing is impossible, causing the saliva to flow out of the mouth, and even breathing is rendered difficult. If the epiglottis becomes enlarged by oedematic swelling, tracheotomy may be necessary, but more often the disease is less grave, pus discharge occurring sooner or being facilitated by early surgical interference, which is possible if the center of the infection can be located.

DIAGNOSIS Local symptoms: The patient complains of the tongue being swollen and too large, of difficulties in swallowing and breathing. If the tongue comes in contact with hard food, it causes a great deal of pain and the saliva often flows from the mouth.

General symptoms: The pulse is generally increased in rate, the temperature rises, and may reach the high marks of septic conditions.

Clinical signs: Examination of the mouth is usually impossible on account of the muscular trismus and the sensitiveness of the tongue to touch. The cervical and submaxillary lymph glands are involved at an early stage of the disease and are extremely tender to touch. Later there is marked angina, causing the patient to bend the head forwards on the chest, which somewhat facilitates the breathing through the nose.

3. *Tubercular Abscesses of the Tongue.*

ETIOLOGY Tubercular abscesses of the tongue may be primary or secondary infections. Tubercular bacilli are found in mouths of healthy persons and primary tubercular infections may therefore occasionally occur at an injured part of the tongue. This, however, is said to be a rare condition. Secondary infection is more common, slight wounds on the tongue caused by carious teeth or sharp artificial dental prostheses are easily infected by the bacilli of the saliva and expectorated material.

CLINICAL COURSE Tubercular abscesses of the tongue occur mostly on the tip, the sides, and the mucous membrane reflection between tongue and floor of the mouth. When first seen they are very small nodules of yellow. A clear infiltration develops, becoming gradually thick and increasingly visible. The lesion usually extends deep into the substance of the tongue, developing a fissure or an ulcer. Tuberculosis fissures are very short, often stellate or branching, and are generally single. The margin is indicated, causing an elevation of the edges which are liable to caseate, forming a foul and ragged surface. The tuberculosis ulcer is the more aggressive form of the fissures and presents edges which are a little thrown up, but not undermined, and are usually sharp in outline. The secretion is small in quantity and is of grayish yellow color. Pale red flesh warts, and here and there small gray knots may be visible.

DIAGNOSIS Local symptoms: Tuberculosis of the tongue is seldom noticed early by the patient, as the lesions first are very small and produce no symptoms; later they become tender and pain becomes pronounced.

General symptoms: The patient may suffer from pulmonary tuberculosis or lupus of the face. However, he may be perfectly well, the lesion of the tongue being a primary infection.

Clinical signs: The appearance of the tubercular lesions of the tongue has already been described. Bacteriological examination of the sputum and excretions is important for making a sure diagnosis. A negative Wasserman test excludes gummata, but carcinoma of the tongue is often difficult to differentiate from tuberculosis with certainty.

II. ABSCESSES OF THE SALIVARY GLANDS AND DUCTS

Abscesses of the salivary glands and ducts may be divided into primary and secondary infections. The sublingual and submaxillary glands are most frequently involved by primary infection, the disease entering through the salivary ducts. The parotid gland is more often the seat of secondary infection, the bacteria entering the gland through the circulation. Salivary calculi are also to be considered. They may either cause or be caused by infection.

ETIOLOGY *Primary Infection.* The primary infection of the salivary glands may be due to a continuous septic process, such as necrosis or ostitis of the mandible, or alveolar abscesses from lower teeth. The pus burrows through the tissue, following the path of least resistance, and often reaches the submaxillary gland, causing Ludwig's angina, a disease which, however, is not restricted to the submaxillary gland, but attacks the muscles of the floor of the mouth and neck. More commonly, however, the infection enters by way of the ducts, originating from pus discharged by sinuses of abscessed teeth, pyorrhoea pockets, or other forms of oral sepsis.

Secondary Infections. Haematogenous infection of the parotid gland is known to occur occasionally after infectious diseases, such as scarlet fever, typhoid fever, measles, meningitis, appendicitis, chalecystitis, and acute abscesses. Any focus causing secondary infection seems therefore to cause disease of the parotid gland and in very rare cases of the other salivary glands.

Salivary calculi. Calculi are more commonly found in the sublingual and submaxillary ducts and glands and are of rather rare occurrence in the parotid gland. The question whether the calculus is primary or secondary to the infection has not yet been entirely settled. The believers in the primary origin of the calculi think that the infection is due to its irritating presence. The men who believe in the infectious origin of the calculi founded their idea upon microscopic investigations. They think that calcium phosphate or carbonate is deposited in concentric fashion around organic exudates as epithelial cells, leucocytes, bacterial emboli, or mucin, or that precipitation of the salts may be due to direct bacterial activity.

Whether primary or secondary, the calculus plays an important rôle in the infections of the salivary glands, and cases which will not yield to treatment and which recur often harbor in their ducts or glandular substance calculi which are a source of irritation and reinfection.

Stones may be found in Stenson's or Wharton's duct or in the body of the glands. They most frequently occur in Wharton's duct and the sublingual gland.

CLINICAL COURSE If the disease starts from the mouth, the infection often does not progress farther than a short distance through the duct. The duct walls become swollen, accumulation of products of infection occurs, and calculi may be formed. Either condition obstructs the flow of saliva. During the time of glandular activity, at meal times, and if tasty food is seen, a tumor like a swelling will occur at the site of the obstruction, causing more or less pain until the duct is sufficiently dilated to allow excretion. Abscess formation usually occurs, discharging either through the duct or forming a new sinus to the mouth.

In ascending duct infections, the process spreads through the accessory ducts, finally involving the glands and interlobular tissue. In the parotid gland the abscess may point towards the face, the mouth, the external auditory canal, or may extend upwards into zygomatic fossa. In the submaxillary and sublingual gland, the abscess will break either to the mouth or through the floor of the mouth to the skin of the submandibular region or the neck. The salivary fistula occuring in this fashion is extremely difficult to heal and often can be closed only by radical surgical procedures.

In the secondary infections the bacteria are carried to the glands in the blood stream and the abscess starts in a blood vessel and progresses to the adjacent parts.

DIAGNOSIS Local symptoms: The patient usually complains of marked swelling in the region of the gland which may frequently change its size. If the duct is affected, the swelling becomes especially marked during glandular activity. If the abscess and stone lie

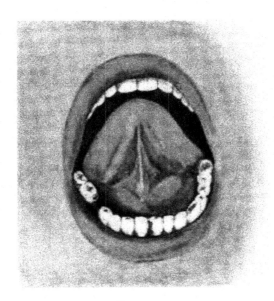

Fig. 113

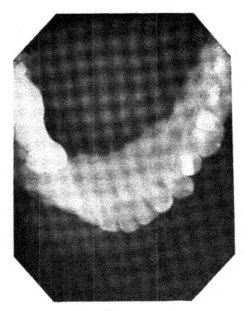

Fig. 114

Fig. 113.—Swelling under the tongue on the left side.
Fig. 114.—Radiograph showing salivary calculus causing
the condition indicated in the picture above.

in the substance of the gland, the swelling is usually of a more inflammatory nature. At times, due to some unknown factor, probably renewed bacterial activity, there are sudden reactions and the patient complains of intense pain. Such attacks occur at irregular intervals and cause a large amount of suffering.

Clinical signs: During the attacks, we usually find the characteristic symptoms of acute abscess formation with more or less swelling of the neighboring tissue, which is not alone due to the accumulation of saliva in the gland, but to oedematic infiltration, especially so in streptococcic infection. The corresponding lymph glands are enlarged, soft, and tender in acute conditions, hard and solid in cases of longer standing, which have passed more or less into a chronic stage. There may be discharge of sero-purulent material through the inflamed orifice of the duct or a fistular bidigital palpitation and careful exploration of the duct with a fine silver probe may reveal a stone, but if the trouble is harbored in the gland itself, this method of diagnosis will be found unsuccessful.

Radiographic examination: Radiographic diagnosis is of greatest importance in glandular affections. Extra-oral, as well as intraoral films, are of greatest value; they not only tell us whether there are calculous obstructions, but also give us their location, a helpful aid for the operating procedure. For sublingual calculi and stones in Wharton's duct, a large film may be placed between the patient's teeth, the head being bent in an extreme backward position so that the rays can be directed from the submandibular region vertically on the film. Submaxillary calculi may be taken by the same method or by placing a film or plate under the mandible, more towards the diseased side, reaching farther back than the angle of the jaw. The picture is taken from above with the mouth wide open.

The treatment of the abscesses of the tongue and salivary glands will be found in the general chapter of treatment of abscesses.

CHAPTER VI

BACTERIOLOGY OF ORAL ABSCESSES

IMPORTANCE OF THE BACTERIOLOGICAL STUDY The careful scientific study of the bacteria found in oral abscesses requires a great deal of time and patience on account of the many varieties which normally inhabit the mouth. These may become the direct cause of abscesses or inhabit the lesions accidentally, living upon the products of decomposition. It is especially the cultivation and isolation of the anaerobic bacteria which renders the investigations difficult. No one has been able to demonstrate that one type of bacteria causes one typical form of dental abscess and it has generally been accepted that any one of the pyogenic bacteria may cause abscesses in the mouth. It has been observed and demonstrated that it is not so much the variety of the bacteria which determines the course of the disease but that it depends upon the number, vitality, and virulence of the invading organisms and, moreover, upon the abundance or scarcity, as quality of the media; such as organic matter in the root canal, whether an abscess will develop as an acute or chronic condition. But also secondary invasions of bacteria and the different combinations of mixed infections determine slight changes in the pathological picture, such as the production of gases, odor of the exudates, and color of the pus. The variations, however, are so manifold and the bacterial causation so accidental that a study of the bacteriology of the dental abscesses was found a fruitless task, and furthermore, an undertaking of small practical importance, until lately, when the process of focal infection was discovered. The bacteriological question, then, becomes at once one of first importance, if we look at the

PLATE XXVI

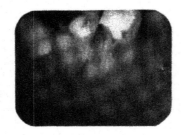

Fig. 115

Fig. 116

FIG. 115.—Radiograph, showing granuloma from which the smear below was made.

FIG. 116.—Microphotograph of a smear taken from abscess seen in Fig. 115. Note the two chains of streptococci and groups of staphylococci.

Specimen prepared by author; stained with methylen blue.

unfilled root canal containing remnants of diseased pulp, or the acute and chronic dental abscess and the granuloma as a focus from which not only bacteria may become absorbed and distributed to other parts of the body, but where protein poisons (see Chapter I) may be generated and taken up by the circulation, thus causing general toxemia or local disease of certain delicate tissues. We have already seen that the protein poisons which are formed during infection differ, among other things, according to the species of the invading bacteria and it is therefore desirable to know which of the bacteria encountered in these lesions produce secondary disease, either by direct infection or by the formation of pathogenic poisons which become absorbed and may cause auto-intoxication similar to that of intestinal origin.

The study of the bacteria of dental abscesses, which was first undertaken to find the etiological factor of the local lesion, has now become of new importance, but from a different reason, namely: that of investigating the effect of pathogenic or saprophytic bacterial life in a certain part of the body called a focus such as a root canal, abscesses, or granuloma upon other parts of the body.

From Acute Abscesses. Wash the mucous
METHODS OF membrane thoroughly with a mild anti-
COLLECTING septic mouth wash (the spray may be
BACTERIAL used). Apply iodine on the gum, and as
SPECIMEN soon as the incision is made, introduce a
sterile pipette deeply into the abscess to collect the pus. The pipette is then sealed and sent to the laboratory. Instead of the pipette a sterile syringe may be used.

From Chronic Abscesses and Granulomata of Teeth which are Extracted. First of all remove the tartar or other deposits from the tooth and spray the mouth and teeth with an antiseptic solution, then scrub the mucous membrane in the region of the offending tooth as carefully as possible. Pack sterile gauze on either side of the tooth to exclude saliva, dry the mucous membrane with gauze and compressed air, and saturate tooth and gum with tincture of iodine. The ligamentum circulare is then cut free from the tooth, after which iodine is employed a second time to destroy bacteria which always lodge immediately under the mucous membrane. Extract the tooth and place the forceps holding the tooth on a piece of sterile gauze, apex of the tooth uppermost. Curette with a sterile instrument the alveolar socket from which the tooth was extracted to remove the granulations, and smear some of the removed tissue over the slant surface of a culture tube. Two plantings may be made, one for aerobic, the other for anaerobic cultures. Immediately after the operation clip off the apex of the removed tooth with sterile Rongeur forceps and drop it into another culture tube. It is advisable to let it drop into the water of condensation and smear it afterwards over the surface of the media.

From Chronic Abscesses and Granulomata in Apiectomy. As this operation is performed under the principles of asepsis no further precautions need to be taken. The amputated root is at once dropped into a culture tube held and opened by an assistant. Other cultures are made from the removed granulation tissue.

METHODS OF BACTERIAL STUDY *Immediate Microscopic Examination.* Pus gained from acute abscesses may be examined directly under the microscope by making the usual cover glass preparations. Also, from chronic condition may we secure cover glass preparations by smearing the end of the root or a piece of infectious granulation tissue over the cover glass.

Inoculation of Artificial Culture Media. Specimens gained from acute or chronic abscesses by the methods already described may be inoculated on artificial media for special identification, and pure cultures may be made of the bacteria which perhaps have already been recognized in a general way in a cover glass preparation.

The cultures should be grown on various media and both under aerobic and anaerobic conditions. Anaerobic bacteria are especially hard to cultivate and it is of greatest importance to inoculate the media without loss of time so as not to endanger the vitality of the anaerobes.

Inoculation of Animals. The animals which are ordinarily used for inoculation are rabbits, guinea pigs, and mice. Rabbits and guinea pigs are usually inoculated by the subcutaneous or intraperitoneal method. A very simple method in rabbits is the intravenous inoculation. The tip of the ear is held by thumb and fingers of the left hand, while the right manipulates the syringe. The needle is pushed through the skin on the external surface into the posterior vein which runs along the margin of the ear. By the exercise of care and gentleness the animal may thus be inoculated without being anaesthetized or even held by an assistant, especially if the fur between its ears is stroked for a short time.

Animal inoculation is used to find out whether the bacteria in question are pyogenic or not. The animal usually dies of the same disease that was produced in man. If bacteria taken from a questionable focus produce in the animal the same disease the patient suffers from, we can conclude that we have found the organism which causes the systemic disease.

REVIEW OF THE BACTER- IOLOGICAL STUDY OF ORAL AB- SCESSES *Schreier** (1893) gives in his article the results of nine examined cases. In five cases he took his material from the inflamed periosteum, involved by an alveolar abscess, and in four cases from a subgingival parulis. In three cases he found only the diplococcus pneumoniae, in three cases only the staphylococcus pyogenes albus, in the remaining three cases he found both the diplococcus and the staphylococcus present. He concludes from this that periostitis (acute abscess) is due to infection by pus producing bacteria and especially to the diplococcus pneumoniae, which, he adds, was also found in two abscesses due to caries examined by Nannotti*; Miller and Sieberth contest that Schreier's diplococcus is identical with the diplococcus pneumoniae.

---

* *See* Bibliography.

Schreier 1893	Diploc. pneumoniae	Staphylococc. p. albus
Case 1.	+	
Case 2.	+	
Case 3.	+	
Case 4.		+
Case 5.		+
Case 6.		+
Case 7.	+	+
Case 8.	+	+
Case 9.	+	+
Nannotti 1891		
Case 1.	+	
Case 2.	+	

*Miller** (1894) examined two cases of alveolar abscesses and found in one two different varieties, in the other one variety of a coccus.

*Arkövy** (1898) examined four cases of periostitis alveolaris chronica diffusa (chronic alveolar abscess, as a sequel to the acute alveolar abscess) and found in one case the bacillus gangraenae pulpae alone, in two cases together with the staphylococcus pyogenes aureus and albus, and in another case there was no growth on the culture plates.

Arkövy 1898	Bac. gangraenae pulpae	Staphylococc. p. aureus	Staphylococc. p. albus
Case 1.	+		
Case 2.	+	+	+
Case 3.	+	+	+
Case 4.			

*Goadby** (1903) pronounces the cocci as the bacteria found in almost all the alveolar abscesses. He examined twenty cases and very often finds a staphylococcus de-

* See Bibliography.

scribed under the name of staphylococcus viscosus. The staphylococcus he finds in half of the cases, the staphylococcus aureus in three cases, and sometimes also the micrococcus tetragenus. In two cases with fetid pus he discovered the bacterium coli and in four cases of diffuse alveolar abscesses he grew besides the staphylococcus albus a constant anaerobic bacterium which formed long threads and produced much gas. When stained with methylen blue it took the color irregularly. He was not able to get a pure culture. This is the first mention of the discovery of an obligate anaerobic microörganism in a pathological process of dental origin.

*Partsch** (1904) reports a well observed case of tuberculosis of the jaws near the apex of a root and for the first time described the microscopic picture of a tubercular periodontitis.

*Monier** (1904), a Frenchman, was the first to make a study of the anaerobic bacteria in connection with his bacteriological study of six alveolar abscesses. In *Case VI,* a boy of the age of nine, who was suffering with *"ostéo-périostite"* (alveolar parulis) caused by a carious left lower first molar he found a micrococcus and a bacillus by microscopic examination and gram stain of the lightly fetid pus. On the surface of agar cultures fine gray colonies grew, which he identified as streptococci. In the depth of the agar cultures where there is exclusion of air he found longitudinal and round granular colonies which he identified as the bacillus Ramosus. In *Case VII,* a woman at the *hôpital *Saint-Antoine,* the following diagnosis was made: *Ostéo-périostite, abscès bien collecté, overture* (large alveolar parulis with sinus) on the left superior or lateral incisor. Microscopic examination of the very liquid, fetid, grayish pus shows leucocytes in the stage of destruction scarcely stained. He found gram positive micrococci of small number and a gram positive bacillus; besides these a gram negative bacillus. Aerobic cultures yielded a scarce growth of streptococci and in anaerobic cultures he found the bacil-

* See Bibliography.

lus fragilis in large quantity and the bacillus Ramosus in small numbers. *Case VIII* he saw in consultation at the *"hôpital de l'Institut Pasteur"* with *"Ostéo-périostite du maxillaire inférieur avec oedéme considérable* (alveolar parulis, with large oedematic swelling) caused by a right lower bicuspid. The abscess broke during the examination; he found streptococci, staphylococci albi, and numerous anaerobic bacteria, among them the bacillus Ramosus. As the material could not be collected with the necessary precautions, the study of this case was not further followed up. *Case IX* was a patient who suffered from an enormous swelling in the submaxillary region, extending over the whole cheek, suborbital region and subhyoid region caused by a tooth in the left lower jaw. There was intense trismus, the skin was covered with an erysipelitic reddish color. During the night there was delirium, the swelling became fluctuating in the submaxillary region and an opening was made with thermocautery. Examination of the horribly fetid pus showed partly destroyed leucocytes and a veritable mixture of microörganisms. He found bacilli of fine and short form often encapsulated, V-shaped bacilli, cocci in chains, and a rare bacillus occurring in filaments. Cultures yielded a streptococcus, bacillus Fragilis and Ramosus which were most abundant; the other unnamed bacteria could also be obtained in pure culture. *Case X,* patient with *"abscés volumineux de la voûte palatine"* (palatal alveolar parulis) from a right upper incisor tooth. The pus which was mixed with black blood showed on microscopic examination only fragments of leucocytes which hardly stained. The enormous quantity of bacteria consisted of diplococci, curved bacilli, often of the shape of a V, which were gram positive, a short and fine bacillus and a rare bacillus of very large form, both gram negative. Inoculation on the surface of agar yielded no growth whatever, but the anaerobic bacteria were very abundant. He isolated the bacillus Fragilis, the curved bacillus which was identified as bacillus Ramosus and the

* See Bibliography.

diplococcus which was found to be the coccus foetidus. The large bacillus which was seen in small quantity grew in large white, coarse cultures and was found to be a bacteria that had not yet been described. This case is interesting because a large amount of pus was produced in this abscess without the presence of any aerobic bacteria but was due to four anaerobes. *Case XI*, a young girl at the *"hôpital des Enfants-Malades,"* had suffered with a great deal of pain from a left inferior first molar for three months. The abscess broke first into the mouth and later formed a sinus to the outside of the face. Microscopic examination of the abundant pus showed well stained leucocytes, and gram positive curved bacilli sometimes occurring in chains of two. Surface cultures stayed sterile but in the middle, deprived of air, he obtained cultures of the bacillus Ramosus, which was the only microörganism found.

MONIER 1904	AEROBES	ANAEROBES				
	Streptococci	Streptococci	Diplococci foetidus	B. Ramosus	B. Fragilis	Undescribed bacilli
Case VI	+			+		
Case VII	+			+	+	
Case VIII				+		
Case IX	+			+	+	+
Case X		+	+	+	+	+
Case XI				+		

*Vincent** (1905) writes in his article *"La symbiose fusospirillaire ses diverses déterminations pathologique"* that he found seven times in seventeen cases of *"suppuration dentaire sous periostique"* (subperiosteal parulis) the association of fuso spirillae, once as a pure infection.

*Mayerhofer** (1909) thinks the streptococci are the primary cause of *"periostitis dentalis"* (alveolar parulis). In examining twenty-two cases of pus gained from unopened abscesses and twenty-eight cases of pus taken

* *See* Bibliography.

from sinuses on the gum, he found thirty times streptococci in pure culture, fourteen times streptococci and
bacilli, twice streptococci and staphylococci, once staphylococci and bacilli, twice stapylococci alone, and once bacilli alone. He thinks that staphylococci are perhaps
present only on account of secondary infection of media
prepared by streptococci and that the bacilli are etiolog-
ically without importance.. Apparently he made no
attempts to grow anaerobes.

MAYERHOFER 1909	STREPTOCOCCI	STAPHYLOCOCCI	BACILLI
30 cases	+		
14 cases	+		+
2 cases	+	+	
1 case	+		+
2 cases		+	
1 case		+	+

*Idman** (1913), of the Pathological Institute of the
Helsingfors University (Finland), has written the most
complete and thorough bacteriological study of the acute
alveolar abscess published in the *"Arbeiten aus dem
Pathologischen Institut der Universität Helsingfors."*
His publication is based upon most careful and painstaking research work, each analysis representing four weeks
of steady, tedious work.

He described his method of obtaining and inoculating
the culture, the preparation of the fourteen different
media used and the staining methods for coverslip examination.

He examined eight cases of undoubted dental origin
which had not undergone therapeutic treatment at any
time, contamination from the fluids of the mouth was
carefully excluded, and by careful technique, the pus was
aspirated by a Pravaz syringe and emptied into a sterile
test tube. The different media were inoculated as soon
as possible, never later than an hour was allowed to elapse,

* *See* Bibliography.

so as not to endanger the vitality of the anaerobes. The oxygen tolerating bacteria were grown on agar (Titer 15-18), blood agar and glucose agar (Titer 15-18). The obligate anaerobes were gained by shake cultures in series of 10-12 tubes of Agar (Titer 2-3), 10-12 tubes of glucose agar (Titer 15-18), 10-12 tubes of ascites glucose agar (Titer ca. 8) and 10-12 tubes of Indigo-glucose agar. Some of the isolated bacteria he tested as to their virulence by subcutaneous inoculation into rabbits or guinea pigs, using 5-10 c.c. of a young bouillon culture. To study the microörganisms gained in these cultures he used gram stain, the polychrom-methylen-blue-tannin method, and Ziehl's carbofuchsin stain.

Case A. A woman thirty years of age, with subgingival parulis, caused by a suppurating pulpitis. The thick yellow pus was of neutral reaction and odorless. Microscopic examination and cultivation showed an oxygen tolerant streptococcus and bacillus mesentericus and obligate anaerobes identified as a streptococcus, Bacillus Ramosus and Idman's bacillus No. 13.

Case B. A nineteen year old peasant boy presented a subgingival parulis from a putrescent pulp. The pus which showed a slightly alkaline reaction, was odorless. The bacteria he isolated were the oxygen tolerant streptococcus, staphylococcus albus, micrococcus tetragenus and the elongated cocci Idman No. 6, the obligate anaerobes, bacillus ramosus. Case C was a patient presenting a subperiostal parulis from a first molar. The yellowish white pus was of extremely fetid odor and slightly alkaline. Cultivation and isolation yielded the oxygen tolerant corynebacterium pseudodiphtheriticum and the obligate anaerobic streptococcus anaerobicus, bacillus ramosus, bacillus thetoides, bacillus perfringens. Case D, a young man, age seventeen, with subperiosteal parulis. Microscopic examination of the exudates showed an abundant bacterial flora which were cultivated and identified as follows: Oxygen tolerant; streptococcus, bacillus Idman* No. 3, obligate anaerobic; streptococcus,

* *See* Bibliography.

staphylococcus parvulus, bacillus ramosus, bacillus thetoides, bacillus perfringens, bacillus bifidus communis and bacillus Idman No. 14. Case E, also a case of subperiosteal parulis with thick yellowish pus without odor nor reaction yielded the oxygen tolerant bacillus Idman No. 3 and the obligate anaerobe bacillus ramosus. Case F, a case of subperiosteal abscess, contained thin pus of strongly alkaline reaction. The following bacteria were found: oxygen tolerant; streptococcus, obligate anaerobe; staphylococcus iungano, staphylococcus parvulus, bacillus thetoides, bacillus ramosus and bacillus fusiformis. Case G, a subgingival abscess with grayish white pus of neutral reaction, contained large oxygen tolerant cocci single, double and in packs, (staphylococci) also small oxygen tolerant streptococci. The obligate anaerobes were found to be streptococci and the bacillus ramosus. Case H, a subgingival abscess, was not fully completed. It contained oxygen tolerant staphylococci and the bacillus ramosus.

IDMAN 1913	OXYGEN TOLERANT							OBLIGATE ANAEROBIC.								
	Streptococci	Staphylococci	Diplococc.	Micrococc. tetragenus	B. mesentericus	B. pseudodiphtherit.	Other bacilli	Streptococci	Staphylococc. Parvulus	Staphylococc. Iungano	B. ramosus	B. thetoides	B. perfringens	B. fusiformis	B. bifidus communis	Other bacilli
Case A	+			+				+			+					+
Case B	+	+	+	+							+					
Case C						+		+			+	+	+			
Case D	+						+	+	+		+	+	+		+	+
Case E								+			+					
Case F	+								+	+	+	+		+		
Case G	+	+						+			+					
Case H		+									+					

PLATE XXVII

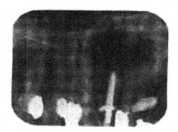

Fig. 117

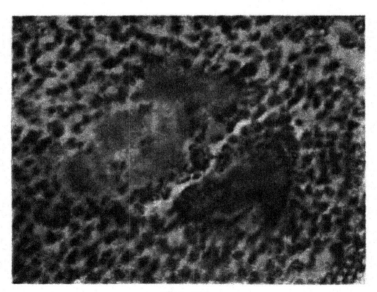

Fig. 118

Fig. 117.—Radiograph of a tooth with large granuloma which proved to contain colonies of actinomyces.

Fig. 118.—Microphotograph of a section of the above granuloma.

Specimen prepared by author; stained with methylen blue and Eosin.

The animal experiments undertaken with these bacteria he reported under a special head, describing the isolated microörganisms.

Bacillus pseudodiphtheriticum (aerobic) was injected into guinea pigs in the form of a 5 c.c. of a 22-hour old bouillon culture. There was an increased temperature on the second day, no other pathological conditions.

Aerobic streptococci, two of which form no haemolysis, two others cause a very weak haemolytic phenomenon, were not all used for animal experiments. One strain of the latter was injected subcutaneously into a rabbit and caused only temporary decrease of weight, but no other pathologic conditions.

Bacillus ramosus (anaerobic) was tested on rabbits. Five of the isolated strains were used, two immediately after the isolation. Ten c.c. of a three to seven days' culture was injected subcutaneously. None produced an abscess at the place of inoculation. In each case he observed a slow decrease in weight lasting from two to three weeks. Only one case resulted in death of the animal after thirty-three days; in all the other cases the animal slowly recovered.

Bacillus perfringens (anaerobic) proved pathogenic for guinea pigs. After injection of 3 c.c. of a fresh bouillon culture an extensive local infiltration occurred which showed, when cut, a foamy oedematic secretion resembling saliva which contained the bacteria in pure culture. With one strain experiments were made to increase the virulence, which was successful after passage through two guinea pigs. The third animal died inside of thirty-six hours after injection of 3 c.c. of a fresh bouillon culture. Culture from the heart blood gave a positive result.

Bacillus bifidus communis (anaerobic) caused no pathogenic effects in rabbits from injection of 10 c.c. of a bouillon culture.

Bacillus thetoides (anaerobic) was used only in one strain for animal experiments. The weight of the rabbits decreased slowly for one week, after which they recovered. Only on the second day there was an increase in temperature.

Streptococci anaerobic, no animal experiments.

Staphylococcus parvulus caused no pathologic conditions in rabbits.

Staphylococcus iungano caused no pathologic conditions after injections of 10 c.c of a bouillon culture.

In regard to these animal experiments, it must be remembered, when compared with the results of Hartzel-Henrici, that the organs of these inoculated animals had apparently not been examined pathologically, and that the pathogenicity of the bacteria was only judged from local effects and as to the life or death of the animal. Hartzel-Henrici observed the low virulence of streptococci infections when injected into animals, producing death only after a long period if at all, although there were serious lesions developing in some of their important organs which can only be demonstrated in microscopic sections of the diseased parts.

*Gilmer** (1914). Gilmer, who reports bacterial examinations of acute and chronic abscesses, in a general way, found streptococci in aerobic cultures, and occasionally the staphylococcus albus and aureus, and the micrococcus catarrhalis. In anaerobic cultures he found streptococci and the bacillus fusiformis either alone or in mixtures, as well as a black pigment-forming organism which usually did not appear for about five days.

*Thoma** (1915). The author reported in a paper read before the American Academy of Dental Science his results of cultures taken since November, 1914, of all abscessed teeth in the hospitals as well as in his private practice. He concludes that any microbes belonging to the flora of the oral cavity may be found in oral abscesses. Streptococci which grew aerobically and anaerobically were found in the majority of cases, sometimes as pure

* *See* Bibliography.

PLATE XXVIII

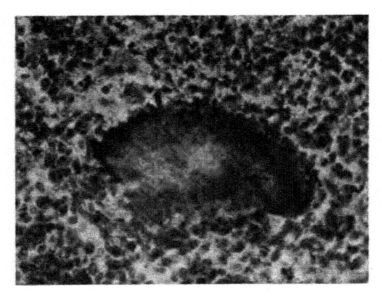

Fig. 119.

Microphotograph of a section of a granuloma containing colonies of actinomyces.

Specimen prepared by the author and stained by the Gram-Weigert Method.

cultures, but frequently mixed with staphylococcus albus and aureus. Besides these he often found an admixture of many other pathogenic and saprophytic bacteria such as the bacillus fusiformis, bacillus coli, the influenza bacillus, and the bacillus proteus.

In two cases he found the fungus of actinomycosis. This organism has been demonstrated several times in root canals by Partsch* and was found by the author in a large granuloma of an upper lateral incisor, and in the root canal as well as in a granuloma of a lower bicuspid of another patient. Both men were city people, there were no clinical symptoms of general actinomycosis of the jaws of soft tissue, which is due to the fibrous encapsulation of the lesion. The first granuloma was removed, by the regular method of thorough curettage used by the author, the character of the abscess was not discovered until later when the specimen, a part of the granuloma, was examined. There was no recurrence of the disease. The other granuloma was adhering to the tooth and the fungus of actinomycosis was found when the specimen was prepared. In order to verify the findings different stains were used, the colonies in the form of rosettes with club-shaped radiating filaments were clearly visible, as seen in Figure 118 and Figure 119.

*Hartzel and Henrici** (1913, 1914 and 1915). The mouth infection research corps of the National Dental Association, consisting of Thomas B. Hartzel, Henrici and Leonard, started in September, 1913, a closer study of "the relationship growing out of the transplantation of the chronic mouth infections to other parts of the body and a study of the areas of inflammation in the human and animal body which have been induced by these transplanted organisms." They were the first who undertook to study systemically the bacteria found in the dental abscesses in regard to their systemic effects rather than as to their etiological local importance. Their

* *See* Bibliography.

bacteriological research work has sought to determine by animal inoculation the character of the damage wrought in the various organs of the body by the introduction of intravenous injections of living organisms cultivated from lesions in the mouths of the patients studied. The bacteriological study reported October, 1914, and November, 1915, in the *Journal of the National Dental Association* alone represents an enormous amount of work and the conclusions drawn from the pathological study of the animal experiments mark a classic epoch in the study of dentistry.

The first report is based upon a study of eighty-two cases, the second report was published after about two hundred additional cases of chronic periodontal infections had been bacteriologically examined. Attention was from two reasons directed almost solely to the streptococci, first because they were constantly present and frequently were the sole cultivable organisms obtained, and secondly, because the research workers made the relationship of dental infections to rheumatism their immediate problem. They however also obtained the staphylococcus albus, the bacillus coli, the bacillus proteus, the bacillus florescens non-liquefaciens and the pneumococcus. Aerobic as well as anaerobic cultures yielded the same results. Cultures made from healthy teeth have constantly been found sterile. The cultural features of the streptococci of these dental lesions then received the writer's attention. On blood agar two kinds of colonies were obtained: "green" colonies, which produced a green halo, and gray colonies without halo. With regard to sugar fermentation reactions for an indicator, for which a beef serum with one per cent. of the various sugars added had been used with acid fuchsin decolorized by potassium hydroxide, they found that the majority of cases ferment either raffinose (streptococcus salivarius) or salicin (streptococcus mitis). Only in one case had a manite fermenter been observed (streptococcus fecalis).

PLATE XXIX

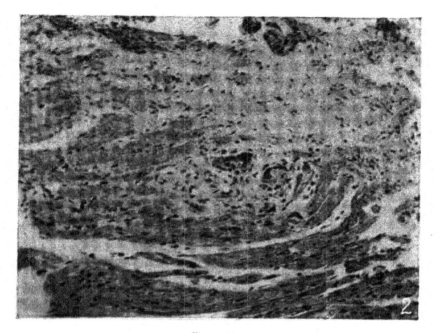

Figure 120.
Chronic myocarditis. The section shows the heart muscle of a rabbit which died 16 days after an injection of streptococci from case No. 55. The section shows an area of fibrosis with several giant cells.

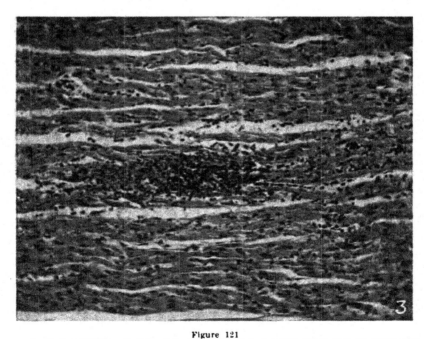

Figure 121
Acute myocarditis. Section of heart muscle from a rabbit which died 48 hours after an injection of streptococci from case No. 60. The section shows an area of lymphoidal infiltration.

Both illustrations reproduced by courtesy of Dr. Hartzel.

TABLE OF FERMENTATION OF STREPTOCOCCI FROM CHRONIC DENTAL LESIONS

No.	Blood Agar	Litmus Milk	Lactose	Saccharose	Mannite	Raffinose	Salicin	Inulin
110	Green	Acid, Coag.	Acid	0	0	0	Acid	0
116	Green	0	Acid	Acid	0	0	Acid	0
121	Green	0	Acid	Acid	0	0	Acid	0
122	Green	Acid	Acid	Acid	0	Acid	Acid	0
123	Green	Acid, Coag.	Acid	Acid	0	Acid	Acid	0
124	Green	Acid	Acid	Acid	0	Acid	Acid	0
125	Green	Acid, Coag.	Acid	Acid	0	Acid	0	0
127	Green	Acid, Coag.	0	Acid	0	0	Acid	0
129	Green	Acid, Coag.	Acid	Acid	0	Acid	Acid	0
130	Green	Acid, Coag.	Acid	0	0	0	Acid	0
133	Green	Acid, Coag.	Acid	Acid	0	Acid	0	0
134	Green	Acid, Coag.	Acid	Acid	Acid	0	Acid	0
135M	Green	Acid, Coag.	Acid	Acid	0	Acid	0	0
135B	Green	Acid, Coag.	Acid	Acid	0	Acid	Acid	0
136	Green	Acid, Coag.	Acid	Acid	0	0	0	0
137	Green	Acid, Coag.	Acid	Acid	0	0	Acid	0
138	Green	Acid	Acid	Acid	0	0	Acid	0
141	Green	0	0	Acid	0	0	0	0
20	Green	Acid	0	Acid	0	0	0	0
21	Green	Acid, Coag.	Acid	Acid	0	0	0	0
23	Green	Acid	Acid	Acid	0	0'	0	0
27	Green	Acid, Coag.	Acid	Acid	0	Acid	0	0
28	Green	Acid, Coag.	0	Acid	0	Acid	Acid	0
29	Green	Acid	Acid	Acid	0	0	0	0
32	Green	Acid	Acid	Acid	0	Acid	Acid	0
34	Green	Acid, Coag.	Acid	Acid	0	0	0	0
35	Green	Acid, Coag.	Acid	Acid	0	Acid	0	0
36	Green	Acid	Acid	Acid	0	Acid	Acid	0

Two facts stand out prominently from their work: members of the streptococcus viridans group are constantly present in chronic dental infections, especially the streptococcus salivarius and the streptococcus mitis, and the common pus-producing haemolytic streptococci are constantly absent.

In their animal experiments they used rabbits exclusively, being more susceptible to streptococci than other laboratory animals. In their first article they describe seven animal experiments from cases which they selected for special research study out of one hundred examined patients. In the second article they mention that they had inoculated two hundred and twelve additional rabbits with twenty-two different strains of streptococci. From these inoculations they are impressed by the comparatively low virulence of these streptococci, though in the end the damage wrought by them in the animal economy was serious and in some instances irreparable. Some of the animals did not die at all, and most died a relatively long time after the inoculation. Of the animals that died, the most striking features were a progressive emaciation and loss of strength. The lesions produced in the animals were of diverse character occurring in the arteries, joints, kidneys and heart. The most common lesions produced were those frequently associated with rheumatism, namely, myocarditis, consisting either of diffuse infiltration of lymphocytes in submaxillary nodules composed of aggregations of lymphocytes or in areas of fibrosis with occasional giant cells. The kidneys were frequently also the seat of disease, consisting of abscesses which contained either polymorphonuclear leucocytes alone or associated with lymphocytes, and which in some cases contained bacterial emboli, or small aggregations of lymphocytes along radial vessels of the medulla. The arterial lesions which occurred occasionally were destructive lesions of the tunica media of the aorta in the ascending portion of the arch with a hypertrophy of the underlying intima.

The hearts, kidneys and large vessels of sixteen healthy rabbits were also examined; no lesions could be found.

The added illustrations have been kindly sent to me by Dr. Hartzel to illustrate this splendid work of his research corps, and I here take one more especial occasion to express my appreciation of his courtesy, which I feel sure will also be greatly appreciated by the interested reader, and induce him to study in detail the important investigations published by Dr. Hartzel and his associates in the various dental and medical magazines.

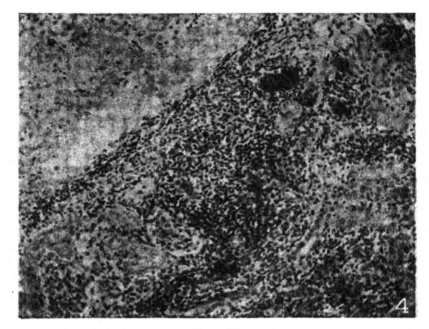

Figure 122
The section shows an area of wide spread infiltration with lymphocytes and poly-morphonuclear leukocytes in the kidney of a rabbit which died 48 hours after an injection of streptococci from case No. 59.   This was the second passage of this streptococcus through rabbits.

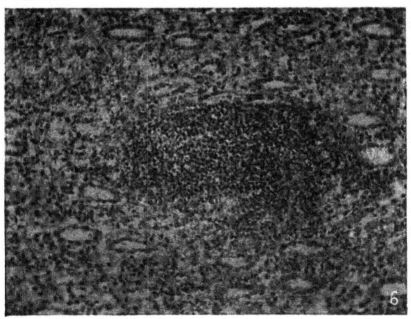

Figure 123
This plate shows a localized polymorphonuclear abscess in the medulla of the kidney of a rabbit which died 48 hours after an injection of streptococci from case No. 60.

Both illustrations reproduced by courtesy of Dr. Hartzel.

Author's Remark.—The investigations of Hartzel and other scientists give the reader the impression that the streptococcus is the only bacteria of the flora found in oral abscesses, which should be seriously considered, and that other bacteria may be looked at, either as contamination or organisms whose activity is restricted to the local lesion. Medical writers also, Rosenow particularly, whose research work has almost revolutionized the etiological theories about certain systemic infectious diseases, considers the streptococcus-pneumococcus group as the causative factor of secondary lesions, caused by transportation from the focus through the blood stream. Amongst the large number of bacteria which may be found in oral abscesses, there are without doubt others which may become absorbed and cause secondary disease or which produce toxins, which when taken into the circulation may affect certain tissues and lower the health of the patient. One of the most commonly found bacteria, besides the streptococci is the staphylococcus. It may be often found alone or together with others. Dr. Steinharter has very recently undertaken bacteria experiments with this organism. While the organisms had not been taken from oral abscesses, I shall nevertheless add an abstract of his experiments, so as to show that other bacteria than the streptococcus group should be considered dangerous to the rest of the body.

Steinharter,[*] 1916. The author published two articles, the first on gastric ulcers, the second on experimental production of acute arthritis by inoculating animals with staphylococcus cultures. Gastric ulcers were produced by injecting an emulsion from the agar growth (prepared by suspending a twenty-four-hour old culture on agar slant in 10 c.c. normal saline) or from the broth (by suspending in 15 c.c. of saline the centrifugal sediment of a twenty-four-hour old 150 c.c. broth growth). One quarter to 1 c.c. of the emulsion was injected with 1 c.c. of a weak acetic acid solution. Forty rabbits were used for the experiments, the hypodermic injections were preceded

* *See* Bibliography.

by a laparotomy, and the post-mortems revealed, if organisms of special virulence were used (for instance, one freshly isolated from the appendix) invariably typical peptic ulcers from one quarter of an inch to one inch in diameter.

Acute arthritis was experimentally produced by injecting intravenously an emulsion, prepared by suspending an agar slant culture in about 10 c.c. of normal saline. The dose used was usually 1 c.c. for a rabbit and 3 c.c. for a dog. It was found that the staphylococcus is apt to localize in the joints and produce typical lesions of arthritis, if the strain is of proper virulence, having a predeliction for this region (staphylococci from joints for example have a decided tendency to again localize in joints) or if the tissue in which the organisms have lodged is suitably altered for their growth and action.

The writer concludes that the staphylococcus may be caused very regularly to localize in the stomach after intravenous injection. It appears that the same organism may be caused to localize in joints and produce typical arthritis. The published protocols show that in some cases arthritis was the only lesion found at autopsy but in other cases it was associated with one or more other lesions, namely duodenal ulcer, appendicitis, cholecystitis, myocarditis, pericarditis, endocarditis, nephritis, colitis and myositis.

PLATE XXXI

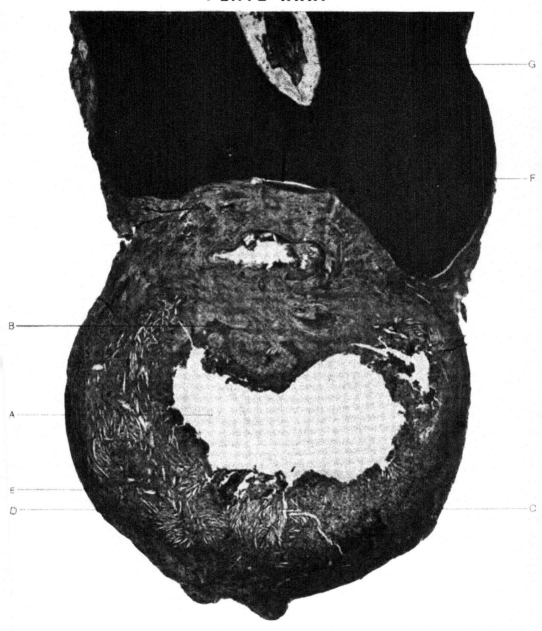

FIG. 124.—Microphotograph of the end of a tooth with an epitheliated granuloma.

A—Lumen.   B—Proliferating epithelium.   C—Cholesterine spaces.
D—Capsule of the granuloma.   E—Blood vessel.   F—Exostosed root end.
G—Root canal.

Stained with Mallory's connective tissue stain.   Specimen prepared by the author.

CHAPTER VII

HISTOLOGICAL PATHOLOGY

The microscopic study of abnormal conditions and disease is not only of great interest to the pathologist, but of far-reaching importance for the understanding of the beginning, progress and termination of disease, as well as of greatest value for the development of the knowledge which furnishes the best foundation upon which intelligent treatment, be it of medicinal or surgical character, may be based.

ACUTE PERIODONTITIS The infection of the periapical tissue of a tooth is transmitted through the apical foramina from the diseased pulp and causes, if the amount and virulence of the injurious agent is right, what is clinically termed as acute inflammation of the periodontal membrane, or acute periodontitis. The reaction consists of circulatory disturbances and inflammatory exudation. The blood vessels, after an initial constriction, become dilated almost to twice their size and leucocytes accumulate along their walls. A serous infiltration with emigration of polymorphonuclear leucocytes occurs which is seen in spaces formed between the fibres of the periodontal membrane. This causes an increase in size of the membrane, pushing the tooth out of its socket and gives the impression of an elongated tooth. If the condition continues, tissue destruction sets in and we find small necrotic areas. This process is most marked near the apical foramina from where the suppuration spreads.

ACUTE ALVEOLAR ABSCESS After a comparatively short time the pus has collected in larger quantity and the bone forming the alveolar socket becomes involved. The fibres of the periodontal membrane still persist, become elongated, and parts of bone are absorbed. While the bone is destroyed the pus cavity enlarges and is called an acute alveolar abscess. If suppuration is very active and prolonged we find destruction of the fibres of the periodontal membrane at the apical part as well as involvement of the cementum of the tooth which shows a necrotic appearance and has been observed to result in loss of more than half of the root of the tooth.

DENTO-ALVEOLAR PARULIS After the destruction of the lamella of the alveolar socket the cancellous part of the bone is freely infiltrated with pus. The Haversian canals are next involved by means of which the pus finds its way through the outer cortical layer of the bone. The periosteal tissue reacts at once causing a local infiltration of polymorphonuclear leucocytes and a widespread serous infiltration causing large oedematic swellings in the cheek and neck. The pus forms first under the periosteum (subperiosteal parulis) which presents a remarkable resistance to the destructive processes of inflammation. After the periosteum has been penetrated, necrosis continues in the submucosa of the gum until it extends to its surface and forms a fistula which gives exit to the accumulated pus.

CHRONIC ALVEOLAR ABSCESS After the process of destruction has reached its climax, nature makes an attempt of healing by the formation of granulation tissue. The necrosed cells are dissolved by the leucocytes and either absorbed or expelled through the sinus. Fibroblasts and vascular endothelium are formed by proliferation to replace the necrosed tissue; destroyed cells and serous or purulent exudation from remaining injurious agents may continue to pass through the newly-formed tissue to the surface. Endothelial leucocytes and lymphocytes may collect in large numbers in the deeper layers of the granulation tissue to counteract the irritating agents absorbed from the exudates. This condition clinically called chronic abscess may last for an unlimited period, the discharge from the fistula may increase at times, if the process of destruction becomes more marked, or may become less or even stop entirely

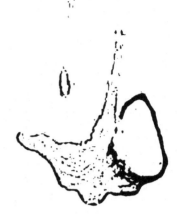

Fɪɢ. 125

Fɪɢ. 125

Fɪɢ. 126

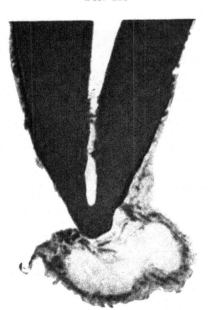

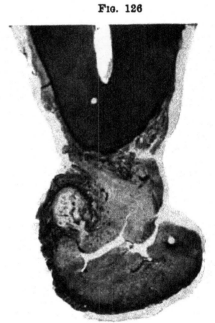

Fɪɢ. 127

Fɪɢ. 128

Fɪɢ. 125.—Microphotograph of a simple granuloma. Part of the pulp has been left in the root canal and the granulation tissue is seen to extend from the root canal through the apical foramen. The blue spot shows a necrosed area in the dentine.

Fɪɢ. 126.—Microphotograph of a simple granuloma showing a distinct capsule. There is necrosis of the root and a lateral lumen.

Fɪɢ. 127.—Microphotograph of a simple granuloma, showing capsule and three places where active pus formation is going on.

Fɪɢ. 128.—Microphotograph of a granuloma with sinus in which pus formation has taken place.

All four specimens were prepared by the author, and stained by Mallory's Phosphotungstic acid, Hematoxylin stain.

for a certain period, a condition which is usually only temporary but frequently brings about the closure of the mouth of the fistula. This will reopen with more or less marked subacute symptoms as soon as the suppurating process has overcome the defense of the body, the process of repair. This picture should impress the importance of removing the cause, viz., a diseased dental pulp or the necrotic end of the root of the guilty tooth. Perfect repair is not possible as long as a necrotic root apex persists.

PROLIFERATING PERIODONTITIS In contrast to the processes of suppuration of the periodontal membrane stands the much more common proliferating periodontitis and its sequels. This is a reaction to mild injurious agents such as bacteria in small numbers and of low virulence, of which the streptococcus mitis and salivarius are good examples and commonly found in these lesions. But also mild toxins or diluted stronger toxins as well as chemicals such as irritating drugs (formaldehyde) sealed in the root canal cause irritation of the periodontal membrane. The reaction occurs first near the apical foramina consisting in a focal accumulation of lymphocytes, an increase in cells and vessels and formation of plasma cells. Endothelial leucocytes and polymorphonuclear leucocytes may be more or less abundant according to the irritating agent causing the inflammation.

DENTAL GRANULOMA The dental granuloma is the sequel of the proliferating periodontitis. Its histological study is extremely interesting. The author has prepared microscopic specimens of about fifty of these lesions in the research laboratory of the Harvard Dental School and the following descriptions are principally based upon original investigations:

Simple granuloma. The new formed tissue gains in size until it has the microscopic appearance of a reddish sack which reaches generally the size of a large pea, but occasionally attains much larger dimensions. The pressure from the growing lesion causes resorption of the

bone and on microscopic examination we find that the
granuloma is surrounded by a fibrous capsule which extends between the trabeculae of the bone.   The fibres of
the encapsulating layer originate from the periodontal
membrane, which in some cases may become detached
from the cementum of the apex, the tooth remaining in
others in a more or less modified way.   The communica-
tions with the root canal usually persist, the granulation
tissue seems to be continuous with remnants of pulp left
in the apical part of the root canal, while at other times
the granulation tissue grows into the root canal.   The
connection between the periodontal membrane and the
peripheral fibrous capsule is often so strong that the
granuloma is removed attached to the tooth in extraction.
In the majority of cases, however, we find that the granuloma remains in the jaws.   The thickness of the capsule
varies greatly and contains fibres, groups of which grow
in various directions.   This fibrous capsule is well illustrated in the microphotographs, Figures 126 and ˋ
127, and in the high-power drawing, Figure 129, stained
by   Mallory's   Phosphotungstic-acid   Hematoxylin
method.   Vessels and capillaries can be seen in all these
illustrations of the fibrous capsule, they are usually surrounded by an increased number of plasma cells and a
small number of leucocytes; their lumen is often greatly
increased, and the endothelial cells often show a proliferating appearance.   Red corpuscles are found in the vessels together with polymorphonuclear leucocytes and a
granular substance.   Such a vessel and capillaries as well
as fibroblasts and infiltrated cells are especially well reproduced in Figure 130, an oil immersion drawing of a
part of the capsule in a section stained with hematoxylin
and eosin.   These studies impress the great attempt
which nature made to wall off the seat of inflammation to
prevent spreading into the neighboring parts.   It, however, also demonstrates that this capsule does not prevent
absorption as it contains a meshwork of capillaries and is
penetrated abundantly by larger vessels and therefore
its contents are in direct communication with the circu-

PLATE XXXIII

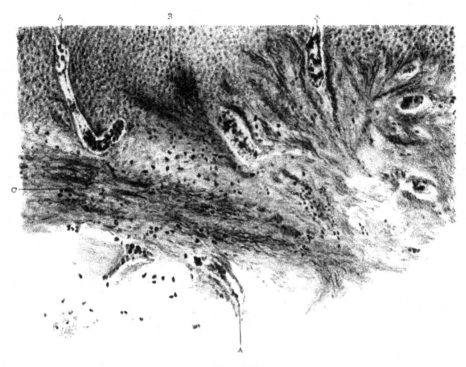

FIG. 129

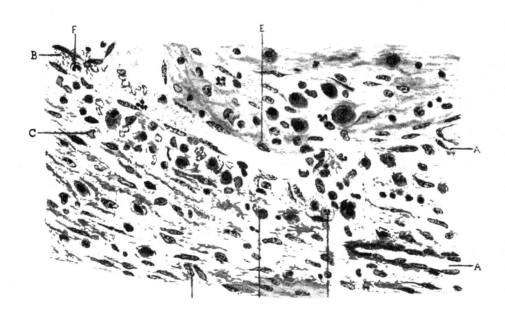

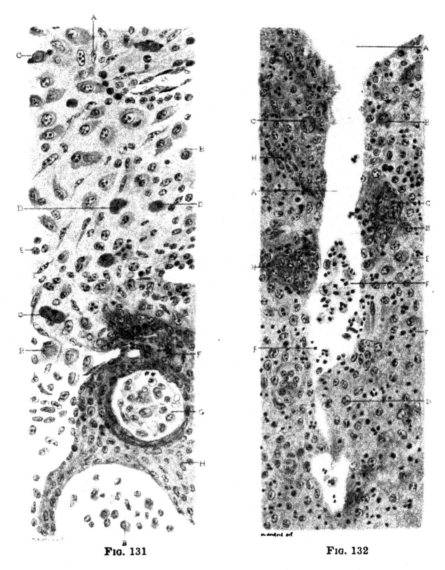

FIG. 131   FIG. 132

FIG. 131.—Lithograph of high-power drawing of epitheliated granuloma as shown in Fig.
124, showing the inner part.

A—Fibroblast. B—Plasma cells. C—Hyalin bodies. D—Eosinophiles. E—Lymphocytes.
F—Leucocytes between epithelial cells. G—Island surrounded by epithelium.
H—Epithelial cells.

Specimen prepared by author and stained with Hematoxylin and Eosin.

FIG. 132.—Lithograph of high-power drawing of the inner part of the granuloma shown in
Fig. 128, showing the upper branch of the sinus.

A—Mouth of sinus. B—Plasma cells. C—Blood vessels. D—Leucocytes.
E—Polymorphonuclear leucocytes. F—Pus cells. H—Epithelial cells.

Specimen prepared by author and stained with Hematoxylin and Eosin.

PLATE XXXV

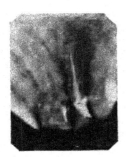

Fig 133

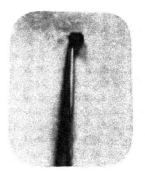

Fig. 134

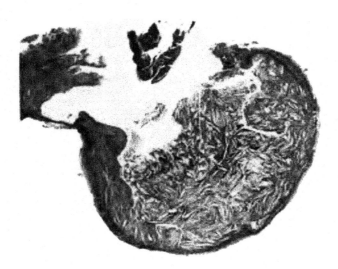

Fig. 135

Fig. 133.—Radiograph showing lateral incisor just after the root canal had been treated and filled. A light circle marks the circumference of the granuloma.

Fig. 134.—Photograph of the same granuloma shown in Fig. 133 after its excision.

Fig. 135.—Microphotograph of granuloma shown in Fig. 133 showing a distinct capsule and numerous spaces which were occupied by cholesterin crystals. Note pink and blue appearance, the first represents fibrin, the second collagen formation.

Specimen prepared by the author, stained by Mallory's connective tissue stain.

lation.   Bacteria and toxins may be absorbed by the capillaries in the granuloma and transported to other parts of the body.   The inner part of the granuloma is made up of granulation tissue (fibroblasts and vascular endothelium) infiltrated by one large mass of plasma cells. These are seen as cells with irregular cytoplasm which has marked basophilic properties containing from one to four nuclei in eccentric arrangement.   If there are processes of retrogression going on we find also numerous polymorphonuclear leucocytes, endothelial leucocytes, lymphocytes, eosinophiles and mast cells abundant more or less.   Erythrocytes are found distributed sometimes throughout the granuloma, at other times only in the fibrous encapsulation; their presence is due to haemorrhage of extended capillaries during extraction.

Epitheliated granuloma.   Remnants of the embryonic enamel organ are commonly found in the normal periodontal membrane of animals as well as man.   They can easily be seen with the microscope and occur either in small groups, islands or in chains.   But the presence of epithelium is not constant in the periodontal membrane, as has been demonstrated by Malassez, and therefore we do not find epithelium in all dental granulomata.   This epithelium may be found only near the root of the tooth in small areas or it may be found throughout the granuloma, having proliferated from the normal remnants, stimulated by the irritating influence of chronic inflammation.   The cells of the proliferating epithelium differ in appearance from the cells of the epithelial islands; they become larger, the cytoplasm and nucleus become more distinct, and leucocytes invade the intercellular substance which loosely connects the various cells.   The epithelial strands are of uneven thickened bands radiating from the original island in various directions, and form when examined in a microscopic section a wide meshwork throughout the granulation tissue.   The epithelium has further the tendency to grow between live and necrosed tissue, and it has sometimes the appearance of encapsulating the seat of suppuration.

Granuloma with Lumen. Suppuration of the simple or epitheliated granuloma frequently sets in either near the apical foramen from where the bacteria emigrate or farther in the center. If the destructive process becomes severe a subacute alveolar abscess results with subperiosteal or subgingival parulis and sinus formation. After the accumulated pus is discharged the symptoms will soon quiet down, but the pus formation may persist in a mild way and discharge through a chronic sinus, as seen in Figure 128. The granulation tissue first shows a large infiltration of polymorphonuclear leucocytes and later areas of necrosis in the center. After a while the pus may be resorbed and if the leucocytic infiltration stops, a lumen remains, containing necrosed tissue. (Figures 124 to 127.)

Besides suppuration we may also find fatty degeneration, especially at the periphery between the fibrous capsule and the granulation tissue. In old conditions there are also other retrograde processes such as the formation of cholesterin crystals, which are recognized by the rhomboid shaped spaces left by the crystals, which dissolve during dehydration in alcohol. They can be demonstrated, however, in frozen section and appear as brownish crystals. Foreign body giant cells frequently surround one or more crystals, as seen in Figure 137. Compare also cholesterin spaces in Figure 124 and Figure 135. Collagen is formed by the fibroblasts from the fibrin which stains blue with Mallory's aniline blue connective tissue stain in contrast to the fibrin and fibroglia fibres which are stained red, as seen in oil immersion drawing Figure 136.

Another retrograde process is the hyalin formation which occurs in droplets of various sizes in the cytoplasm of the plasma cells (Russell's fuschsin bodies). This causes the cells to enlarge and often nothing remains of the cell but the acidophilic hyaline bodies. These are usually diffusely scattered through the whole granuloma.

Cysts. In the epitheliated granuloma with lumen we frequently find an attempt of the epithelium to line the

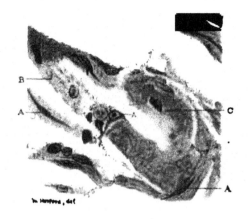

FIG. 136

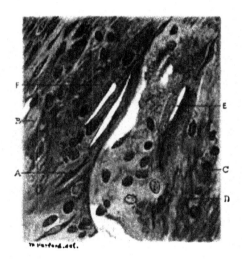

FIG. 137

FIG. 136.—Lithograph of high-power drawing showing the construction of the granuloma shown in Fig. 135.
A, Fibroblasts, with fibroglia fibres. B, Fibrin.
C, Collagen.

FIG. 137.—Lithograph of high-power drawing showing the construction of another part of the granuloma shown in Fig. 135.

A, Fibroblast, with fibroglia fibres. B, Fibrin.
C, Erythrocyte. D, Connective tissue bundles.
E, Space from cholesterin crystal.
F, Giant cell enclosing cholesterin spaces.

central space. This influenced the German writers to call Epitheliated granulomata with lumen formation, "root cysts." Dependorf, in a lengthy article, describes with careful illustrations the formation of cysts from dental granulomata. The author agrees that cysts may be formed in both jaws from such conditions, but this must happen extremely seldom or we would meet with cysts more commonly in these days where granulomata are found in almost everybody's mouth.

CHAPTER VIII

SECONDARY COMPLICATIONS

The acute forms of oral abscesses have always been more or less feared, more because of their violent symptoms than on account of the serious complications which may result if treatment is neglected or if the cause is not removed. The chronic forms, on the contrary, have mostly gone unnoticed, although they occur much more frequently. They were not properly recognized until the radiograph became essential as a means of diagnosis and only recently we became aware of the fact that almost every devitalized tooth develops this condition. In my opinion, it is a fair estimate to say that seventy-five per cent. of the population of this country harbors this lesion in the mouth. In the Robert B. Brigham Hospital for chronic invalids I found that of eighty-two patients, seventy-three suffered from chronic abscesses; some of them also had pyorrhoea, and in the mouths of these seventy-three patients I found three hundred and thirty-four abscesses.

The fact that these chronic abscesses give little or no local symptoms is the reason why the dental profession at large has not been aware of what is going on. But the last few years the deceiving character of these lesions has come to light. Radiographic diagnosis, keen observation and research have revealed the knowledge of the grave consequences of such conditions. These septic foci not only are liable to spread disease to the adjoining parts, but also cause disturbances in organs and tissues quite remote from the teeth.

Continuous Infection. The infection is liable to spread to adjoining parts and involve large areas of the mandibular or maxillary bones, the antrum of Highmore or the throat.

Referred Nervous Irritation. Reflex manifestations from one branch of the fifth nerve to another or to communicating nerves is of quite frequent occurrence, but often such pains are due to the most obscure causes, found only after a most painstaking examination.

Infections through the Alimentary Canal. Abscesses with sinuses or pyorrhoea pockets as well as septic surface lesions of the mouth discharge their pus into the oral cavity where it mingles with the fluids of the mouth and when swallowed reaches the stomach and intestine. The persisting infection through this channel gives rise to most serious diseases of the mucosa of the alimentary canal. From these secondary lesions bacteria may be absorbed into the circulation, in turn causing other diseases by haematogenous infection.

Lymphatic Infection. The lymphatic system and especially the lymph glands have the office of absorbing and disposing of harmful substances, such as liberated in all inflammatory conditions. A certain amount of pus may, however, reach the circulation via the lymph system, while not infrequently we find the lymphatics or the glands seriously affected.

Haematogenous Infection. Abscesses especially of the proliferating type which have no outlet into the mouth, contain, as we have seen, numerous capillaries and blood vessels. Absorption of products of inflammation into the blood stream is usually small in quantity, but constantly wears out the protective cells and causes diseases of the blood and secondary infections in other parts due to transported bacteria, or toxin, or both. The bacteria and products of infection are not only absorbed from the original focus, but also from secondary diseases of the lymph system or the alimentary canal as already mentioned.

The complications which arise from septic foci in the mouth will not be classified in this book according to the mode of infection, but the various disturbances and diseases which have been found due to oral abscesses will be considered in turn. Case reports are here given so as to illustrate the connection of the oral abscesses with the various systemic diseases.

1. *Involvement of Neighboring Parts.*

The inflammation, whether from acute or chronic abscess, is liable to spread to adjacent parts. The spreading to and involvement of other teeth has been mentioned at another place. It has also been explained that necrosis, osteitis, or osteomyelitis is involved in every case of alveolar abscess in a mild and localized way. These diseases may become continuous and involve large parts of the maxillary and mandibular bones if the conditions are right.

MAXILLARY SINUSITIS Maxillary sinusitis or empyema of the antrum of Highmore is very frequently met with by the rhinologist as well as by the oral surgeon. About 75% of the cases are due to dental origin and most are a sequel to oral abscesses.

ACUTE MAXILLARY SINUSITIS Etiology: Acute maxillary sinuses occur only as sequels of nasal or dental diseases. The nasal sources are coryza, influenza, tuberculosis and syphilis of the nasal mucous membrane, and any suppurative process in the nose or other accessory sinuses. Dental sources are acute alveolar abscess on an upper bicuspid or molar discharging into the antrum, infection from a chronic abscess or osteomyelitis in the maxillary bone. Infected dental pulps and root canal instrumentations have been mentioned as etiological factors in cases where the roots project into the antrum. Infection is liable to occur from the extraction of a tooth or root, if a root is pushed into the antrum, or if infected tissue or pus is forced into it and by the introduction of unclean instruments.

Symptoms: The cheek on the infected side becomes reddened and tender, and often there is a marked oedematic swelling which may close the eye. The patient complains of a fullness in the affected side, with a dull throbbing pain, and generally malaise, dizziness, and photophobia. There may be discharge of pus through the nostril, or if the patient lies in bed, into the pharynx. Often the osteum is closed up, when the pain and fullness becomes more marked, and is relieved if part of the pus escapes into the nose. Headaches and neuralgic face-aches are principally found in less severe cases.

Clinical signs: Fever is always present in acute cases and may reach 104°F. An examination of the nares shows usually crusts of pus and congested mucous membrane. In doubtful cases the patient should be asked to sleep on the suspected side and notice in the morning whether there is any discharge upon turning the head to the other side. The patient may be asked to apply suction to the nose while closing the nostrils. Transillumination shows bright illumination under the orbit of the healthy face and darkness on the other. Radiographic examination is the surest means of diagnosis. The diseased antrum presents an opaque appearance on a frontal plate, and a lateral view shows the cause if it is of dental origin. Intraoral films are a great help to diagnose the etiological factor, but are of no value in the diagnosis of the condition of the antrum.

Treatment of Acute Maxillary Sinusitis from the Nasal Cavity. In cases of nasal origin the treatment is undertaken through the nose, but also in certain dental cases this treatment is indicated, especially if the inflammation of the antrum occurs after an extraction, the socket having healed up before the complication sets in.

1. *Irrigation Through the Natural Orifice.* In mild cases, which respond easily to treatment, daily irrigation and medication through the osteum is sufficient.

2. *Perforation of the Nasal Wall.* If drainage and treatment through the natural orifice is not sufficient, perforation of the naso-antral wall with a trocar and cannula is recommended. The opening should be made as near the floor of the antrum as possible. This closes up in a comparatively short time, and resection of a larger part of the wall is recommended if a more permanent opening is desired.

Treatment of Acute Maxillary Sinusitis from the Oral Cavity. It has already been stated that in a large number of cases maxillary sinusitis is due to abscessed teeth. The radical removal of the cause is naturally the first step, but this also furnishes an opening into the antrum through which treatment can be undertaken. The opening is enlarged with the surgical burr and all granulations and diseased bone should also be carefully removed. The antrum is then washed out through the wound by inserting a sterile soft rubber catheter, to which the antrum syringe or fountain syringe is attached. Use lukewarm normal salt solution. If the osteum is closed, spray the antral side of the middle meatus with Sol. Adrenalin hydrochlorid 1:6000. This will contract the mucous membrane and reopen the natural passage way. After the washing has been completed, close the wound with sterile gauze. The washing can be repeated in the same maner until the antrum is healed, when the socket should be closed by a plastic operation. If the antrum is opened accidentally after extraction, and curetting for alveolar abscess, especially if we desire to remove diseased bone, it is advisable to clean first the socket thoroughly and then insert a sterile soft rubber catheter, washing the antrum out as above. Carefully close the wound, and if no reinfection occurs the condition will heal without trouble.

CHRONIC MAXILLARY SINUSITIS Etiology: The chronic form of maxillary sinusitis or chronic empyema of the antrum frequently follows the acute form. Often we find old chronic cases which never were preceded by any acute or painful condition. In these cases granulation is very pronounced and the cavity is filled with polypi. Abscessed teeth play a most important part in the etiology of chronic maxillary sinusitis.

Symptoms: Pain in the cheek, which is often of neuralgic character, is almost always the symptom from which the patient seeks relief. The discharge of pus through the nostril of the affected side is at times very marked and, moreover, it is often of very offensive odor.

The osteum becomes occasionally obstructed, which increases the severity of the symptoms. The patient almost always loses weight. General malaise, arthritis, gastric disturbances from swallowing pus, and mental depression frequently accompany the disease.

Clinical signs: What has been said for the acute condition is also true for the chronic. The differentiation of acute and chronic empyema of the antrum cannot be easily made either by transillumination or by radiographic examination. The history of the case and consideration of the etiological factor will help in ascertaining the condition, but a sure diagnosis can only be made by actual examination. Holmes's naso-pharyngoscope is a great help for this purpose. A short incision in the canine fossa allows us to make an opening through the anterior wall with a surgical burr, through which the naso-pharyngoscope is inserted. The condition of the mucous membrane, the amount and quality of new growth can plainly be seen. This is the safest way of making a differentiating diagnosis.

Treatment: The cause of the disease has to be ascertained and thoroughly removed. Frequently we find cases of maxillary sinusitis which have not improved, although a great amount of time has been spent for treatment. After careful examination we find that a tooth is continuing to reinfect the mucous membrane. To try to save one tooth if two are involved is poor judgment if we consider how difficult a task it is to cure chronic maxillary sinusitis.

There are a large number of methods for treatment of chronic empyema.

Treatment Through the Alveolar Border. The method of draining the antrum through the alveolar process has been in great favor with the dentists. Some have even gone so far as to treat the antrum through the root canal of a tooth. If we compare the small size of a root canal even when enlarged with the capacity of the antrum holding 12 to 52 c.c. of fluid we must see the impossibility of such an undertaking, not to speak of the consideration of that tooth and the infected periapical tissue as a causative factor which ought to be removed. The tooth socket sufficiently enlarged with a surgical burr is the most ideal place for drainage, as it is at the lowest level. The antrum should be washed with the greatest aseptic precautions. A soft rubber catheter can be introduced and is connected either with the fountain or the antrum syringe. I use warm normal salt solution or mild antiseptics as washings, occasionally with application of fifteen per cent. Argyrol. After washing the antrum, care should be taken to remove all the moisture, as the antrum is an air sinus with dry mucous membrane. Frequently I use filtered compressed air for this purpose, administered through the catheter. The washings should be undertaken first daily and later at intervals until there is no discharge for two weeks. It is important to construct a rubber or gutta percha obturator to fit into the alveolar socket principally to prevent food and saliva from entering the antrum, but also to keep the opening from closing up. After the antrum has healed the socket should be closed permanently by a plastic operation.

Operation Through the Canine Fossa. In cases where examination of the antrum reveals granulations and new growth, the foredescribed method is not sufficient to result in a cure. Surgical removal of all growth is indicated. In cases of malignant growth, the lining membrane should be removed radically, but in all cases of polypous and granulating character the tendency is to be contented to remove the growth and not the membrane. A great deal depends in this operation on being able to see all parts of the antrum, and the operation should therefore be performed from the place which gives the best access to vision as well as instrumentation, and this is the canine fossa.

The antrum is opened from the canine fossa by excising the anterior wall with chisel and surgical burrs. The opening should be made large, but care should be taken not to injure the nerves and vessels of the teeth. After the cavity has been freed from polypi, or other

PLATE XXXVII

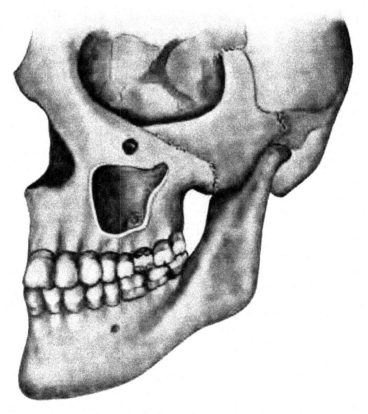

Fig. 138.—Antrum exposed so as to show the abscess formed at the floor by the upper first molar.

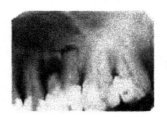

FIG. 139

FIG. 140

FIG. 139.—Radiograph of Case No. 1, showing the condition of the upper first
molar, causing the disease of the antrum.

FIG. 140.—Radiographic plate of Case No. 1, showing healthy antrum (dark) on
the left side of the picture, diseased antrum (cloudy) on the right side.

growth, and from bone septa, the extraction of the involved teeth is undertaken. Chronic abscesses are to be extensively removed and osteomyelitic bone is curetted. After washing out all débris and diseased tissue the cavity is dried out, the alveolar wound closed by sutures, and the antrum packed with antiseptic gauze which should remain in place for about forty-eight hours. Then the gauze is removed, the cavity again irrigated, dried and repacked. This treatment should be continued for about ten days, after which time an obturator, which has been constructed from gutta percha or rubber, is inserted to keep the antrum open for irrigation and observation until it is entirely healed. The plug then can be left out and the antrum is closed by a plastic operation.

Operation Through .Canine Fossa and Treatment Through Nasal Wall. (Caldwell-Luc.) The operation is undertaken through the canine fossa which is closed up immediately afterwards. The after-treatment is then continued through the opening in the antro-nasal wall which is usually of permanent character.

Operation Through Canine Fossa and Treatment Through Alveolar Socket. The canine fossa operation is performed as described, but the alveolar wound is kept open. The opening in the canine fossa is closed after the healing has progressed to a satisfactory stage. An obturator is constructed for the alveolar opening to close the communication of the antrum and mouth after each irrigation. When the condition is cured, the alveolar opening is also closed by plastic methods.

ILLUSTRATIVE CASES *Case I.* (Chronic maxillary sinusitis with polypoid granulations.) The patient, a man of 41 years of age, presented symptoms of chronic maxillary sinusitis. A frontal radiograph is shown in Figure 140, and the cause was ascertained by an intraoral film, Figure 139. The upper first molar shows chronic abscesses on all roots, which apparently infected the antrum. Examination of the nose revealed no infectious condition. Surgical treatment was undertaken by opening through the canine fossa. A large amount of polypoid granulation was found, the antrum was almost entirely filled with it.   I removed the granulations, extracted the tooth and removed all diseased bone with surgical burrs.   The canine fossa was permitted to close after one week, and the treatment continued through the alveolar socket.   After the treatment was completed so that no discharge collected during a period of three weeks, I closed the alveolar opening by a plastic operation.

Case II. (Chronic maxillary sinusitis.) The patient, a man 36 years of age, suffered from obscure pain in the maxillary region.   The two upper bicuspids on the affected side he said had been treated several times, when it was observed that a broach could be pushed up a surprisingly long distance.   An intraoral film showed no extensive periapical condition; a frontal radiograph revealed a slight cloudiness of the antrum.   I opened the antrum from the canine fossa.   Inspection with the nasopharyngoscope showed a condition similar to Figure 138, an antral abscess on the floor over each of the devitalized teeth.   The roots extended into the antrum, and as there was no bone destruction, there was nothing to show in the film.   Extraction of the teeth and curettage of the diseased part was the first step in the treatment, after which the slightly inflamed membrane yielded rapidly to treatment.

PHARYNGITIS Pharyngitis very frequently occurs as a complication of abscesses on lower impacted wisdom teeth.   The inflammation may spread over one side of the pharynx and cause the patient to consult the physician while the real cause is unnoticed on account of lack of symptoms.   (Figure 95.)

Symptoms: Examination of the mouth usually reveals the true character of the condition.   Sometimes the cusp of an unerupted wisdom tooth is visible, and upon pressure on the lingual part of the gum there is usually more or less discharge of pus through the gingival opening.   A radiograph aids sure diagnosis.

Treatment: The cause is to be removed at once.   The pharyngitis should receive general and local attention.

ILLUSTRATIVE CASE *Case III.* (Marked pharyngitis and slight trismus.) The patient, a young man, went to his physician for treatment of the throat. He was referred to me and when he came to my office the next day he had a temperature of 101°F., enlarged maxillary glands on the left side, and slight trismus of the muscles of mastication. On examination of the mouth and pharynx, I found the right side badly inflamed and a large amount of pus discharging from behind the lower second molar. The radiograph showed the cause of the trouble as an impacted unerupted wisdom tooth with extensive abscess formation.

TRISMUS Trismus is a tonic spasm of the muscles of mastication.

Etiology: It is usually caused by an impacted wisdom tooth with abscess formation and periostitis.

Symptoms: The patient complains of not being able to open the mouth except a small distance. Sometimes the teeth are locked in complete occlusion. Pain, inflammation of the pharynx, and swelling of the submaxillary glands are almost always found.

Diagnosis: By means of an extraoral radiograph we are able to determine the cause in a very short time.

Treatment: In mild cases we may use local anaesthesia. After the inferior alveolar nerve and tissues supplied have been anaesthetized in the pterygo-mandibular space by the intra- or extra-oral method, the patient is relieved of pain and usually is able to open the mouth sufficiently for the operation. It is advisable to insert a mouthprop for the patient to bite on. In very severe cases and difficult impactions ether anaesthesia is advisable. The mouth then can be forced open by means of the mouth gag. A few days after the cause is removed the jaw regains its normal function.

ILLUSTRATIVE CASE *Case IV.* (Mandibular trismus.) The patient, aged 24, suffered from pain in the trigeminal region for several days; he also complained of severe earache. He was scarcely able to open his mouth. An X-ray plate showed a right lower third molar which had been decayed and abscessed. The mouth was opened under ether anaesthesia and the tooth extracted. An iodoform wick was inserted for drainage, the patient improved rapidly and was entirely well after one week.

2. *Ophthalmic Disturbances.*

Ophthalmic disturbances due to oral conditions may be brought about in two ways: first, through nervous irritation, and, second, through haematogenous infection.

The ophthalmic division of the fifth nerve, which is purely sensory, supplies the eyeball, the mucous membrane of the eye, the lacrimal gland, and the skin of the brow and forehead. A branch of the second division, the orbital nerve, communicates with the lacrimal nerve; therefore we have direct communication between the first and second divisions. However, the teeth are also connected with the eye through the second and third divisions via the Gasserian ganglion. The first division further communicates with the motor nerves of the eye, the third, fourth, and sixth cranial nerves. Reflex irritation from the oral cavity therefore may not only result in irritation of the parts of the eye supplied by the sensory nerves, but may also cause motor nerve disturbances interfering with the function of accommodation and convergence.

Haematogenous infection, however, here plays an important rôle. To me it seems more probable that secondary ophthalmic disturbances should be of an infectious nature. They may also have been predisposed by reflex nerve irritation. In many cases there may be found a cause in the mouth for referred nervous irritation, but almost always we can also discover a septic focus such as a chronic abscess, an abscess around and caused by an impacted tooth from which the secondary disease may have originated. There is no doubt that oral abscesses as well as oral nerve irritation cause ophthalmic disturbances in many instances, such as iritis, keratitis, scleritis, and

PLATE XXXIX

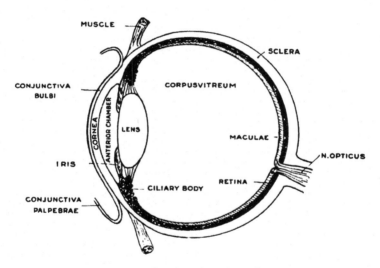

FIG. 141.—Cross section through eye.

PLATE XL

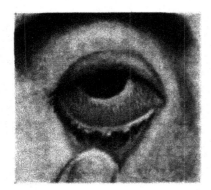

FIG. 142

FIG. 143

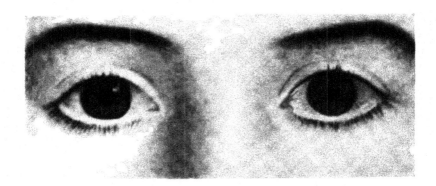

FIG. 144

FIG. 142.—Acute catarrhal conjunctivitis.
FIG. 143.—Simple ulcer of the cornea.
FIG. 144.—Normal eye for comparison and iritis on other side.

All three illustrations are reproduced from May's "Diseases of the Eye," by special permission of the author.

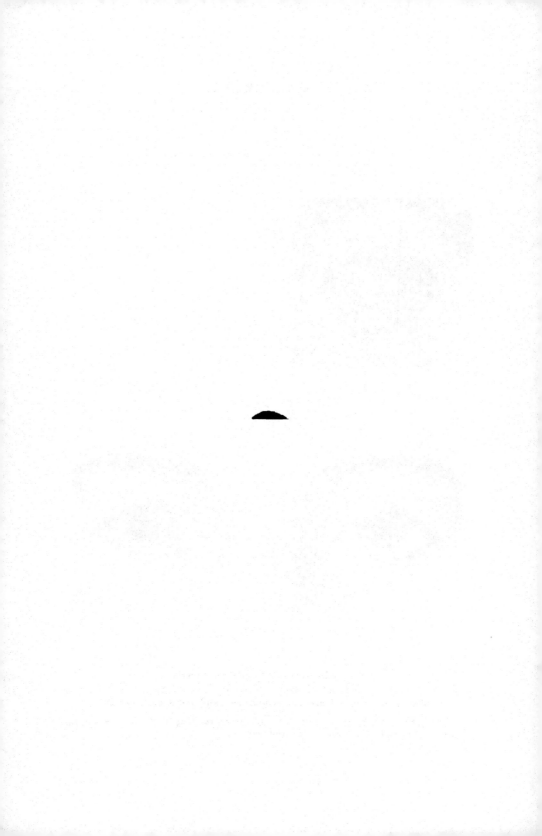

other infectious diseases of the eye, as well as neurotic affections such as intraocular and retrobulbar optic neuritis.

INFECTIOUS CONJUNCTIVITIS Conjunctivitis is an inflammation of the conjunctiva, the thin mucous membrane lining the eyelids. We distinguish palpebral and bulbar types. It is also known as ophthalmia.

Etiology: Infectious conjunctivitis is very often haematogenous in character, but may also be the result of direct contact, as by means of the fingers. It is frequently found in children and may easily be contracted from abscessed temporary molars if the child carries the finger from the aching tooth to the eye.

Symptoms: The conjunctiva is of a brilliant red color and is swollen. The discharge is mucopurulent, sometimes causing blurring of the sight. There are itching and smarting sensations referred to the lids, which feel hot and heavy.

SUPPURATIVE KERATITIS The inflammation of the cornea is called keratitis.

Etiology: It is a process of infection caused by various organisms. It may come from conjunctival inflammations or other direct and indirect infections.

Symptoms: It begins with a dull, grayish or grayish-yellow infiltration of a circumscribed portion of the cornea. It may extend in area and in depth. There is pain, photobia (intolerance to light), lacrimation (excessive secretion of tears), and often blepharospasm (excessive winking).

SCLERITIS The inflammation of the sclera, which with the cornea forms the external tunic of the eyeball, is called scleritis.

Etiology: Scleritis is often seen in connection with rheumatism, syphilis, and tuberculosis. Exposure to cold is sometimes an exciting cause. Reflex irritation and secondary infection from oral foci are not uncommon causes.

Symptoms: There is usually slight discomfort, lacrimation and pain.

ILLUSTRATIVE CASE *Case* V. (Bulbar conjunctivitis.) The patient, a young man, about twenty-two years old, had suffered for a long period from bulbar conjunctivitis of both eyes, for which he was treated by a competent ophthalmologist, who, however, was not able to cure the condition permanently. The two upper central incisors had been devitalized and in the radiograph showed areas of lessened density around their apices. After each subacute attack of these abscesses he suffered from an attack of conjunctivitis. The root canals of both teeth had previously been treated, but the left tooth did not yield to treatment. I treated and filled the left incisor and immediately performed apiectomy.. The patient was normal for about four months, when he had a recurrence. The right eye, which formerly was the worst, showed only a slight conjunctivitis; the left eye was moderately inflamed. The right central incisor again felt lame. I undertook at once to take radiographs of his whole mouth and found a devitalized right lower bicuspid, with slight periodontitis and poor root-canal filling. A right upper bicuspid showed an area of decreased density. Upon opening into this tooth the eye on the same side cleared up almost immediately. The tooth was treated twice with ionic medication and then filled with the chloroform-resin-gutta-percha method. The left eye stayed inflamed, the inflammation also extended into the conjunctiva and did not improve until the root of the right central incisor was amputated. A small granuloma was removed with the root end, which yielded a streptococcus and staphylococcus albus. Three days after the operation, when the patient came to my office for the removal of the sutures, his eyes showed a clear and healthy appearance. Before this case is dismissed apiectomy will be performed on the devitalized upper and lower bicuspids.

IRITIS Iritis is the inflammation of the iris, and may be acute or chronic; primary if developing in the iris itself, secondary if the inflammation spreads from neighboring parts, such as the cornea.

Etiology: Iritis is frequently dependent upon some constitutional disease and therefore may be caused by haematogenous infection. Frequently the focus is found in the nose or mouth.

Symptoms: There is pain, photobia, lacrimation, and interference with vision. The iris appears swollen, dull, with indistinct markings. The color changes and becomes greenish to muddy according to the color of the eyes.

CYCLITIS Iritis is frequently associated with cyclitis which rarely occurs alone. (Iridocyclitis.) It is an inflammation of the ciliary body and almost always involves the choroid.

Etiology: The various causes of iritis are responsible for iridocyclitis. "The disease," writes May, "is often due to the influence of toxins of bacterial origin derived from the teeth (abscesses and pyorrhoea alveolaris) tonsils, pharynx, nose, and sinuses."

Symptoms: In iridiocyclitis we have the symptoms of iritis and in addition tenderness in the ciliary region and often swelling of the upper lid.

CHOROIDITIS Choroiditis may be non-suppurative or suppurative. In the latter case there is usually an involvement of the ciliary body and the iris. It is then called iridochoroiditis.

Etiology: The condition may be of ectogenous or endogenous origin. The latter is due to septic infections from the oral (abscesses pyorrhoea) and nasal cavities, from intestinal autointoxication, syphilis and tuberculosis.

Symptoms: In pure choroiditis there are no external signs; the symptoms are disturbances of sight. In iridochoroiditis there are symptoms of iridocyclitis which are acute and severe.

RETINITIS The inflammation of the retina is called retinitis.

Etiology: Retinitis occurs occasionally as a local lesion, but almost always is a manifestation of a constitutional disease, autointoxication or secondary infection.

Symptoms: Diminution of acuteness of vision is usually present. Pain is rare and there are no external signs.

INTRAOCU-LAR OPTIC NEURITIS In this type of optic neuritis the head of the optic nerve is affected, causing marked visible changes in the disc. Intraocular neuritis is also called *Papillitis*.

Etiology: Among the causes of this disease we have secondary infections from diseases of the nasal cavity, the sinuses and the mouth and teeth.

Symptoms: Disturbance of vision varies and there may be complete blindness. There is no pain and no external signs.

RETROBULBAR OPTIC NEURITIS Retrobulbar optic neuritis involves the orbital portion of the optic nerve, the process being an interstitial neuritis. It may be acute or chronic.

Etiology: It may be due to direct extension from the orbit, general diseases or haematogenous infection. Oral sepsis plays an important part in the latter factor.

Symptoms: In the acute form there is severe headache on the affected side, pain in the orbit aggravated by movement of the eye and rapid impairment of sight, beginning in the center of the field. In the chronic type there is diminution in acuteness of sight, foggy vision, especially in bright light, and blindness in the center.

ILLUSTRATIVE CASE *Case VI.* (Retrobulbar optic neuritis.) The patient, a young woman, was sent to me by an ophthalmologist of this city, with the following letter: "I treated Miss —— some three or four years ago for an acute retrobulbar optic neuritis of each eye. At that time we could trace no cause for the process. About ten days ago, Miss —— developed the same trouble again in her left eye. It is a coincidence that both at the time of this attack and at her previous attack she was having trouble with her teeth. I am sending her to you to get an opinion as to what sort of condition her teeth are in and as to whether there might possibly be an infection there responsible for the ocular trouble."

The patient complained of blurred vision; she was almost blind for near sight, but vision for distance was

PLATE XLI

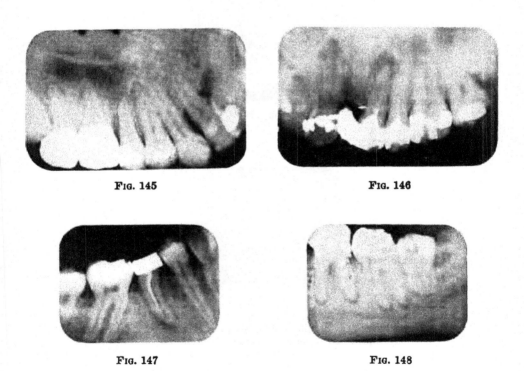

FIG. 145

FIG. 146

FIG. 147

FIG. 148

FIGS. 145, 146, 147 and 148.—Radiographs of Case No. 6, a patient suffering of a retro-bulbar optic neuritis. Both maxillary third molars are impacted. Areas indicating granulomata are found on devitalized teeth.

PLATE XLII

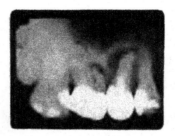

FIG. 149

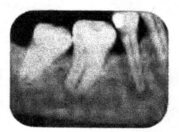

FIG. 150

FIG. 149.—Radiograph showing impacted unerupted third molar causing otitis media in
Case No. 7.

FIG. 150.—Radiograph showing lower second bicuspid with decay under filling and granuloma
causing otalgia in Case No. 8.

not bad. Upon examination of the mouth several poorly-fitting gold crowns were visible. Radiographic examination revealed the following (Figures 145 to 148):

Lower jaw: All the molars of the left side showed areas which indicated chronic abscesses. A very large area on the right second bicuspid.

Upper jaw: Third molar unerupted and impacted on both sides. Left upper first and second bicuspid and right upper first bicuspid, first and second molars also had apical infections to a greater or less extent.

I extracted all these teeth, curetted thoroughly and treated the sockets with iodine. The patient reported improved ten days later, and since then has been steadily growing better.

GLAUCOMA Glaucoma is an important and common disease of the eye which has for its characteristic an increase in intraocular tension. It may be primary or secondary.

Primary glaucoma occurs without antecedent ocular disease, and is divided into inflammatory or congested acute and chronic stages and into non-inflammatory or simple varieties.

Secondary glaucoma is the name given to cases of increased tension and other symptoms of glaucoma due to some other ocular diseases or injuries.

Etiology: The exact cause of primary glaucoma is unknown. May thinks that arteriosclerosis, cardiac diseases, chronic constipation, the gouty and rheumatic diathesis are predisposing factors, all diseases which are more or less caused by toxic or bacterial absorption.

Symptoms: There are different stages distinguished in acute inflammatory glaucoma. The prodromal stage: Sight appears to be obscured by a fog, with slight pain in eye and head. The active stage of glaucoma (glaucomatous attack) is characterized by rapid failure of sight, severe pain in the eye and violent headache, accompanied with nausea, vomiting, and general depression. After a few days or weeks, a decided improvement takes place, but the normal condition does not return. This condition is the glaucomatous stage. At any time there may be new attacks and with each succeeding attack the diminution in vision becomes greater until blindness ensues. This stage is called absolute glaucoma. Later the eyeball is apt to degenerate.

Chronic inflammatory glaucoma is much more common, the symptoms resemble those just described, but are less intense and more gradual in onset. The termination is absolute glaucoma and finally degeneration.

3. *Aural Disturbances.*

Pain in the ear is a very frequent symptom of oral diseases, both the second division of the fifth nerve which supplies the upper teeth and the third division which supplies the lower teeth being in communication with the nerves of the ear. The maxillary division is connected with the tympanic plexus via spheno-palatine (Meckel's) ganglion, the vidian and greater superficial petrosal nerve. The mandibular division communicates with the tympanic plexus by way of the optic ganglion and the small superficial petrosal nerve.

OTITIS
MEDIA
Such irritation of the middle ear referred through nervous channels frequently predisposes the tissue for infection and through haematogenous transportation of bacteria may result in acute median otitis as well as chronic purulent inflammation of the middle ear and tympanum. Abscessed teeth may become foci for purulent otitis in two ways: first, by discharging a large amount of pus into the mouth, which may reach the tympanic cavity via the Eustachian tubes. It is well known that middle ear inflammations occur most frequently in children at the time when they are about to lose the temporary teeth, which very often are badly neglected and abscessed. The pathogenic connection between teeth and middle ear has, however, not alone been demonstrable in children. Grayson reports that in adults he has failed a number of times to

PLATE XLIII

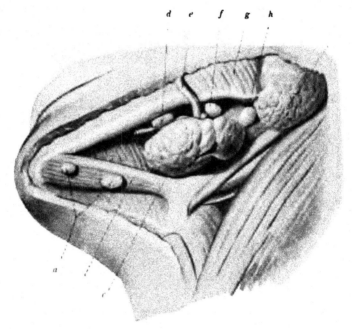

FIG. 151.—Position of the lymph glands beneath the lower jaw (Preiswerk).

a, Submental lymph glands. *b*, Digastric muscle. *c*, Submaxillary gland. *d*, *f*, *h*, Submaxillary lymph glands, A, B, C. *e*, External maxillary artery. *g*, Masseter muscle. *i*, Parotid gland.

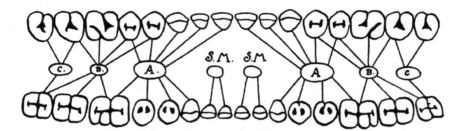

Fig. 152.—Schematic drawing showing which teeth are drained by the various lymph glands.

A, B, C, the three submaxillary lymph glands.
S. M., S. M., the submental lymph glands.

make much impression upon chronic purulent inflammations of the tympanum until the dental cause had been removed.

OTALGIA Otalgia or pain referable to the ear may be from the Pinna, the external auditory meatus, the tympanic membrane, the tympanic cavity, and Eustachian tubes, from the mastoid process, or a reflex manifestation.

REFLEX OTALGIA The jaws and teeth play a most important rôle in reflex otalgia. The pain may be continuous or periodical, with remissions and exacerbations. The cause may be found in the molar region, usually more in the lower than in the upper jaw. Impacted teeth, teeth with acute or chronic abscesses, periostitis, and wounds in that region play a great part as etiological factors.

ILLUSTRATIVE CASE *Case VII.* (Otitis media.) The patient suffered from repeated attacks of otitis media of the right ear. There was a large amount of discharge from the ear. Treatment did not result in permanent relief, and pain persisted after the inflammation had subsided. The specialist she consulted during her last attack in San Francisco, before she left for the East, advised her to have her teeth examined. The patient was then referred to me, and I immediately took radiographs of her mouth. There was a large area over the right upper second bicuspid, shadows on each of the roots of the first molar and a badly impacted upper wisdom tooth with pus discharge from an opening in the gum. I extracted the upper second bicuspid and first molar and extirpated the impacted third molar without disturbing the second molar. The granulomata were removed at once, after which the bone was thoroughly curetted. Local conductive anaesthesia was used for the operation, which also relieved the pain in the ear while it was in effect. During the after treatment the patient improved rapidly and was freed from the aural pain and inflammation. (Figure 149.)

Case VIII. (Otalgia.) The patient, a young lady, referred to me by another patient, complained of earache on the right side; occasionally also had what she called faceache on the same side. She consulted two dentists, who failed to locate the cause of the trouble, and was about to go to an ear specialist when her friend, who had a similar experience, the cause of which I was able to locate and remove, advised her to consult me first. I took radiographs of the teeth on the affected side, and found that the right lower second bicuspid had a large obscure cavity at the distal side, underneath the cervical margin of a gold filling. The pulp was involved and a granuloma had developed at the end of the root. There were no symptoms that indicated this condition. The tooth was extracted and the bone curetted, which resulted in permanent relief of the otalgia. (Figure 150.)

4. *Lymphatic Infections.*

There are two groups of lymph glands which drain the jaws and teeth and their mucous membrane. The submental glands take care of the region of the lower incisor teeth. They are situated behind the chin, beneath the fascia, and between the two geniohyoid muscles. The other group are the submaxillary lymph glands. They are three in number. The anterior one lies internally to the lower border of the mandible and anterior to the external maxillary artery. It is connected with the region of the superior incisors, cuspids, and bicuspids, also the lower cuspids, bicuspids and the lower first molars. The middle submaxillary lymph gland lies posterior to the external maxillary artery at the anterior part of the submaxillary salivary gland. It drains the parts containing the maxillary first molar, but also partly the upper bicuspids and second molar. In the lower jaw it takes care of the three molars, but principally of the second molar. The posterior gland is situated at the posterior pole of the submaxillary salivary gland and is connected with the upper wisdom tooth exclusively, and also with the lower third molar, which is to small extent drained by the middle gland.

These just described lymph glands are tributaries of the deep cervical lymph glands which accompany the external and internal jugular veins.

In a perfectly normal condition these glands are of very small size so that they are hardly noticeable; they are seldom larger than the size of a pea, but in diseased condition they may become greatly enlarged. Lymphatic infections occur most frequently in children, but are not a rare occurrence in adults.

LYMPHAN-GITIS Lymphangitis is an inflammation of the lymphatic vessels, and also gives rise to inflammation of the tissue immediately surrounding them. It is rarely a primary condition and usually extends from the focus to the nearest lymphatic gland, but may continue from there to the next group of lymph glands.

Etiology: The cause is always a septic condition. It occurs in the mouth occasionally from abscesses or other infections. The bacteria or their toxins are absorbed from the focus and cause inflammation while passing along the lymph channels.

Symptoms: We can easily recognize a lymphangitis by the pink or reddish colored streaks clearly visible on the skin. There is usually more or less pain along the lymphatic vessels and a rise of the temperature. Lymphangitis from lesions in the mouth is only recognizable if the lymphatic channels beyond the submental or submaxillary lymph glands are affected, in which cases there is also swelling of these glands. The affection therefore does not point directly to the lesion and the cause has to be ascertained by radiographic examination. The affected gland, however, indicates the location of the focus.

Treatment: The finding and removing of the cause is imperative and if this is done the inflammation will disappear in a short time. Hot applications can be applied as soon as the focus has been thoroughly opened and drainage established.

ILLUSTRATIVE CASE *Case IX.* (Lymphangitis.) The patient, a woman of middle age, presented a lymphangitis extending from the left submandibular region to the left axilla and breast. The lymphatic channels were distinctly outlined in reddish color. The submaxillary and cervical glands were slightly enlarged and tender on pressure. No pain in the mouth. Radiographic examination revealed a large area of lessened density around the left lower second bicuspid. (Figure 153.) Examination showed slight swelling on the gum and pus discharge at the gingival margin if pressure was applied. The treatment consisted in extraction of the tooth, thorough curettage, and insertion of iodoform wick for drainage. This was changed until the discharge stopped and then left to heal up. Bacterial examination showed a streptococcus and staphylococcus aureus infection. The inflammation of the lymphatics gradually diminished and disappeared entirely after three weeks.

LYMPHA-DENITIS Lymphadenitis is the term applied to the inflammation of the lymph glands. We distinguish acute, chronic, and subacute lymphadenitis. Submaxillary, submental, and cervical adenitis are common complications of diseased teeth, especially in children, and unfortunately it occurs frequently that the glands are removed without investigating the unsuspected cause, which almost always is an acute or chronic abscess, from a temporary, permanent, or impacted and unerupted tooth.

ACUTE CERVICAL LYM-PHADENITIS Acute lymphadenitis usually occurs in connection with acute periodontitis and acute abscesses.

Etiology: Acute lymphadenitis is usually secondary to a septic infection. The focus for the submaxillary and submental lymph glands may be found in the orbit, zygomatic and temporal fossae, the nose, the cheeks, palate, lips and especially the alveolar process and teeth of both jaws. Alveolar abscesses and stomatitis are the most

PLATE XLV

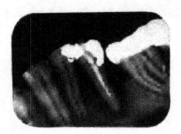

Fig. 153

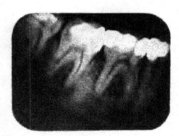

Fig. 154

Fig. 153.—Radiograph showing the tooth (second bicuspid) causing lymphangitis of Case No. 9.

Fig. 154.—Radiograph showing the lower second molar causing lymphadenitis in Case No. 10.

FIG. 155

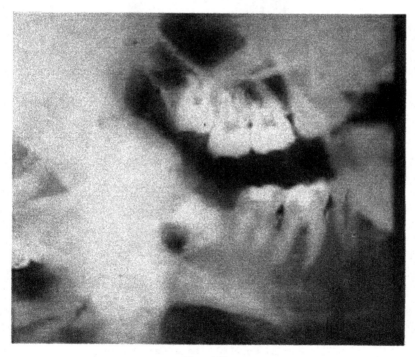

FIG. 155a

FIGS. 155 and 155a.—Radiographic plates of Case No. 11, showing the unerupted third molars causing chronic lymphadenitis. There was a
considerable amount of pus about these teeth.

frequent causes. The toxins or bacteria themselves may be absorbed.

Symptoms: The glands in acute lymphadenitis become only slightly enlarged, they feel elastic and soft, and are very sensitive on palpitation. But also the tissues surrounding the glands become affected by the process of inflammation, the skin looks red and swollen, and in extreme cases the pus may burst through the capsule of the gland and force its way through the skin.

Treatment: Find and remove the focus and use cold poultices and hot mouth wash until the abscess in the mouth has healed, then apply hot poultices to the glands. If suppuration has progressed beyond the stage where nature can take care of the condition, the glands should be incised.

ILLUSTRATIVE CASE *Case X.* (Acute Lymphadenitis.) A young man, a medical student, consulted me for tenderness directly under his lower jaw. Upon examination, I found the middle lymph gland of the right submaxillary group slightly enlarged and very tender; there was also enlargement of one or two of the cervical glands. The examination of the mouth revealed nothing except large amalgam fillings in the posterior teeth. I took a radiograph of the right lower molars first, and was at once rewarded in finding a large area of lessened density extending from the roots of the right lower second molar. A radiograph of the upper molars showed all teeth in normal condition. The pulp of the right lower molar had never been touched before, but apparently was infected. The reason why there were no other symptoms was probably due to the thickness of the outer and inner plate of the mandible in this region, not allowing the pus to penetrate quickly to the large cancellous inner portion, allowing the pus to accumulate without causing pressure or pain. When I opened into the pulp, I found what I expected, namely, an extremely putrescent pulp. After the local condition was treated, the glands became normal in a very short time. (Figure 154.)

CHRONIC CERVICAL LYMPHA- DENITIS If the lymph glands are swollen and remain so on account of persistent infection for a long time, we have chronic lymphadenitis.

Etiology: Chronic lymphadenitis is a secondary infection. It is caused by continuous absorption, such as bacteria from chronic abscesses or pyorrhoea.

Symptoms: The glands are usually much larger than in the acute condition. They are hard, are easily palpitated, and are not tender on touch. They are not adherent and seldom suppurate.

Treatment: The focus should be removed because there is always danger of a secondary infection such as tuberculosis, reaching the gland via the primary lesion.

SUBACUTE CERVICAL LYMPHA- DENITIS Subacute lymph glands occur from subacute attacks in the primary lesion.

Symptoms: Besides the symptoms caused about the focus, we find the lymph glands very large and extremely tender. This is characteristic for subacute attacks.

Treatment: The treatment is the same as for the acute condition.

ILLUSTRATIVE CASE *Case XI.* (Chronic lymphadenitis.) A young lady of about 18 years, was sent to me with radiographs showing four impacted wisdom teeth. She complained of swellings in the submaxillary region, which from time to time became very tender and painful. On examination the gums around the wisdom teeth are found red and inflamed, discharging pus on pressure; the posterior submaxillary lymph gland on each side is much enlarged. I extracted all four impacted teeth under ether anaesthesia, and after the wounds had healed the glands diminished gradually to their normal size. (Figure 155.)

TUBERCULAR CERVICAL LYMPHA- DENITIS Tubercular cervical lymphadenitis is more frequent in children under six years, but is not a rare occurrence in adults. That it occurs independent of general tuberculosis due to septic infection from the mouth was shown by Professor Cantani in fifty clinical observations at the Institute of Medical Clinic of the Royal University of Naples.

Etiology: The cause is the tubercle bacillus, which may find its way to the glands via the lymph system or circulation from the tonsils or the teeth. Carious teeth with open pulp chambers are an ideal place for the entrance of such microörganisms.

Symptoms: The glands first are enlarged and firm, and it is characteristic that in a short time other glands are involved and the structures in the vicinity of the glands become fused together. (Peri-adenitis.) It is also characteristic that the swelling of the glands does not go back after removal of the focus. In cases where the infection is secondary to tuberculosis of the lungs, bones, etc., the glands do not become excessively enlarged, but in primary infections we have large glands which tend to break down.

Treatment: The treatment more or less depends on the question whether the patient suffers from general tuberculosis or whether the cervical lymphadenitis is only a local infection. If the patient's general health is poor, it should be improved by outdoor life and plenty of good nourishment. In treating local conditions we should ascertain and radically remove the cause. Radiographic examination is necessary to ascertain abscesses resulting from teeth, because chronic abscesses give no symptoms or signs to indicate the condition. The removal of the cause, however, does not cure a cervical tubercular adenitis and many treatments have been advised for this condition.

Extirpation: Surgical removal according to many writers is not justified in cases of moderate size because they claim that tubercular adenitis is liable to recur. I think the reason for the recurrence may rather be found in the neglect or insufficient treatment of the cause than in the method. However, it may be advisable to try one or more of the other methods before resorting to radical means.

Heliotherapy: This treatment consists in exposing the glands to direct sunlight.

Radiotherapy: A series of X-ray treatments has been found to give good results. The X-rays are carefully filtered to prevent burning and the dosage is regulated according to the patient and the condition. About twenty treatments applied twice a week are said to be sufficient. This treatment is also advised in cases where suppuration occurs. The abscess may be punctured if a sinus does not already exist. X-ray treatment is also beneficial after extirpation to prevent recurrence.

Injections of Antiseptics: Injections into the glands of iodine or carbolic acid have been advocated. De Vecchis, an Italian physician, has used the following method which had not failed him in a single case, and has the advantage of not causing a permanent scar or fibrous thickening, which fact is important from an aesthetic viewpoint, especially in women. After careful search for and removal or treatment of the focus or possible foci in the mouth and throat, he injects the following solution:

Synthetic guaiacol Merck.........	6.0
Metallic iodine	3.0
Sodium iodid	6.0
Glycerine	30.0
Saccharin	0.5
Aqua dest	10.0

Mx et solve.
Sig. for injections.

With needles of special size he makes parenchymatous injections with this solution, turning the needle in all directions in the gland and liberating the drug drop by drop, using 1 to 2 c.c. in all. The injection is followed by slight massage and by application of tincture of iodine and warm cotton for twenty minutes. When suppuration has begun, he aspirates all pus-like liquid, and if the patient can be seen daily, he also uses gluteal injections of 1 c.c. each day. In regard to the parenchymatous injections the operator should be particularly careful in regard to asepsis, so as not to cause mixed infection. After each injection the gland becomes more tumid, warmer and more reddish, but after one or two days it begins to diminish in size. The injection is repeated twice a week for three to four weeks; the patient is directed to use an antiseptic mouth wash and gargle, to avoid smoking and drinking of intoxicating beverages, and is advised to live in the fresh air and sleep with the windows open, to eat as much as he can of the most nutritious food.

ILLUSTRATIVE CASE *Case XII.* (Tubercular lymphadenitis.) (Case reported by Stark in *Revue de la Tuberculose,* July, 1896.) A youth who had always been healthy previous to his eighteenth year, developed at that age enlarged glands. Carious molars were present on both sides. The glands were removed and the teeth extracted. The glands proved to be tuberculosis and the cover slip preparations from the teeth revealed tubercle bacilli.

5. *Diseases of the Alimentary Canal.*

The mouth and teeth have a very close relation to the rest of the alimentary canal both in health and disease. There are three ways in which digestive disturbances occur.

1. *Insufficient Mastication.* The mouth is the place where the food should be properly prepared for digestion by crushing it into small pieces and mixing it with saliva. A full set of teeth, especially bicuspids and molars, is necessary to accomplish this. Lack of chewing surface, sore and carious teeth or malocclusion mean imperfect mastication, and consequently increased and unnecessary work for the stomach. "While such a condition leads to various ills connected with impaired digestion," says Hunter, "it is not the most important relation of dental diseases to general health."

2. *Swallowing of Bacteria and Pus.* Most serious gastric and intestinal disturbances are liable to result from continuous swallowing of pus and bacteria, which are either mixed into the food during mastication or

reach the stomach between meals. Oral diseases producing such conditions are numerous and common, oral abscesses discharging through sinuses into the mouth, stomatitis and pyorrhoea are of greatest importance. Ill-fitting crowns and fixed bridges, which often cause most contaminating unsanitary conditions, are also a source of gingival inflammation and ulceration.

The discharge from these diseased conditions is continuously taken into the stomach. For a long time the acids of the stomach have been looked at as destructive to such bacteria, but Smithies,* in a microscopic examination of gastric extracts from 2,406 different individuals with "stomach complaint," showed that irrespective of the degree of acidity of such gastric extracts, bacteria were present in eighty-seven per cent. Hunter says there is a limit to the power of the stomach to destroy such organisms. Even in health it is never complete and is solely due to the presence of free HCl. But these powers become progressively weakened, when through any cause an increased and continuous supply of pus organisms is associated with a diminished and continually lessening acidity of the gastric juice. During the intervals between digestion the acidity of the stomach reaches normally a low level which also gives bacteria a good chance to live and multiply in the stomach.

These conditions lead eventually to deeper seated changes in the mucosa of the stomach, and also pass through into the intestinal tract. They pass through the small intestine, where they also may enter into the blood stream to the large intestine where they may exist in large numbers. In this fashion enteritis, colitis and appendicitis may be caused.

3. *Haematogenous Infections of the Alimentary Canal Due to Oral Foci.* Rosenow† writes that hemorrhages, superficial erosions and definite ulceration of the mucous membrane of the stomach and duodenum occur in man not infrequently during severe infections. He produced

---

* Cited from Mayo: Mouth infection as a source of systemic disease.

† ROSENOW: The production of ulcer of the stomach by injection of streptococci.

ulcers in the stomach or duodenum, or both, of eighteen rabbits, six dogs, and in one monkey by intravenous injections of certain streptococci, which have a certain grade of virulence.

SEPTIC GASTRITIS Many writers describe only acute and chronic catarrhal gastritis and mention bacterial infection invading the stomach from the nose and accessory sinuses, the throat and oral cavity as one of the causes. Hunter, however, distinguishes a septic gastritis due to pyogenic infection of the stomach. The term acute and chronic is principally used to indicate a case which is temporary in its course or of a case which shows little tendency towards spontaneous recovery.

Etiology: Professor Miller already recognized the fact that indigestion may be associated with foul mouth, and he brought a charge against the physicians that "their custom of disregarding dental diseases altogether as a factor in pathology is as unjust to their patients as it is discreditable to their profession."

Septic gastritis is caused by continuous swallowing of pus organisms such as are discharged from oral abscesses with sinus and pyorrhoea pockets, infected tonsils or septic diseases of the nose. Not all these bacteria are destroyed, as has already been explained, and the mucosa becomes eventually infected, a septic catarrh is set up which is continuously sustained by influx of pyogenic bacteria.

Symptoms: Clamminess of the mouth, distaste of food, coated tongue and bad taste in the mouth are not so much manifestations of gastric catarrh as the direct result of oral sepsis. The real symptoms are indigestion, gastric discomfort, and nausea.

ILLUSTRATIVE CASE *Case XIII.* (Subacute gastritis.) Reported in Hunter's "Pernicious Anemia," page 231.) A lady, aged sixty-two years, suffered from subacute gastritis. The patient had severe intermittent sickness and gastric pain of eight months' duration, necessitating the use of morphia, with loss of weight and increasing weakness. Cancer was suspected, but on examination no sign of malignant disease was found in the stomach, the abdomen, the rectum or the uterus. Constant complaint was made of a bitter taste in the mouth, nausea, with loathing and distaste for all food. The tongue was coated with a dirty moist fur. The patient had false teeth both in the upper and lower jaws. The plates were scrupulously clean, and the gums beneath the plates were perfectly healthy. There were four remaining teeth, three of them decayed, suppurating around the roots, with pus welling up on pressure. There was no other sign of disease. A provisional diagnosis was made of gastritis caused by continual swallowing of pus. The roots were ordered to be extracted. A week later, the tongue was clean, the sense of taste returned for the first time for eight months, and there had been only one attack of pain. In another week, there was a return of the sickness, with vomiting on pain and slight fever. The vomit obtained two weeks later was watery, with rusty flakes consisting of mucous, fibrin, catarrhal cells, leucocytes and blood, the whole being loaded with streptococci, staphylococci and a few bacilli. A diagnosis was made of infective (septic) gastric catarrh. As a local antiseptic, three grains of salicylic acid were given thrice a day, with peptonized milk as food; counter irritation was applied. There was complete cessation of all pain, and a steady recovery from that time onward. The patient gained weight rapidly and has since remained well (two years).

SEPTIC ENTERITIS Similar to septic gastritis Hunter distinguishes a special form of the disease, namely, septic enteritis, which is in his experience a very common result of prolonged oral sepsis.

Etiology: The bacteria which continuously enter the stomach and escape destruction naturally find their way into the intestine, where they finally infect the thin epithelial layer of the mucous membrane.

Symptoms: There is more or less abdominal pain and diarrhea containing undigested food and mucous, whitish in color, and sometimes semi-solid.

ILLUSTRATIVE CASE

Case XIV. (Case of Enteritis.) Dr. Hunter's case reported in the *British Medical Journal,* November 19, 1904, page 1361. The patient, aged thirty-seven. Foul oral sepsis; most intense gastritis, enteritis and colitis, chronic renal disease, pericarditis, uraemia. Patient died, and microscopic examination of the stomach showed: intense gastritis with invasion of mucosa by masses of streptococci.

APPENDICITIS COLITIS PROCTITIS

The bacterial invasion descends along the alimentary canal and may cause appendicitis, colitis and proctitis. The appendix is predisposed to infection on account of its poor blood supply (appendicitis is most commonly caused by the bacillus coli, the staphylococci and streptococci). Haematogenous infection is also supposed to cause appendicitis, Poynton and Paine have caused it experimentally in rabbits with the organism isolated from rheumatic cases. If the colon is involved, the disease is called colitis, and if the mucous membrane of the rectum becomes infected, we speak of proctitis.

GASTRIC AND DUODENAL ULCERS

Rosenow's work shows that in gastric and intestinal ulcers the mucosa is attacked from behind through the blood stream. It is therefore a disease due to haematogenous infection.

Etiology: The bacteria causing these ulcerating conditions are supposed to have a selective affinity for these particular areas. Predisposing factors, however, may have a good deal to do with the localization of the disease. Clinicians have observed aggravations of symptoms in ulcer of the stomach following sore throat, and the association of these conditions with septic foci in the mouth have been emphasized by various writers. Experimental evidence has been furnished by producing ulcers when injecting bacteria into the gastric artery by Rosenow's experiments on rabbits, dogs, and monkeys with the streptococcus. Steinharter* produced gastric ulcers experimentally in rabbits by injecting staphylococcus cultures

* *See* Bibliography.

of a special virulence and a weak acetic acid solution into the wall of the stomach. In the forty animals used for the experiments typical peptic ulcers were produced varying from one quarter of an inch to one inch in diameter. He concludes: "In the light of the above results, it seems possible that the staphylococcus is responsible for certain cases of gastric ulcer in human beings. If by some means (through an erosion or trauma, etc.) a hyperacid gastric juice enters the tissues of a limited area of the stomach, wall, and if the staphylococcus of proper virulence finds lodgment there, it does seem quite probable that the necessary conditions used in producing the experimental ulcer would be duplicated.

Symptoms: About the first symptom of intestinal ulcer is the occurrence of pain lasting for an hour or two after the ingestion of a hurried meal, or after the taking of food that needs unusual activity of digestion. Hyperacidity and over-secretion, vomiting, and hemorrhages are other symptoms of this disease. The blood may be found in the vomitus or stool.

ILLUSTRATIVE CASE *Case XV.* (Gastric ulcer.) (One of the cases reported by Hartzel in the *Journal of the National Dental Association,* November, 1915, page 341.) The patient, a laborer, thirty-one years of age, of Irish descent, weighing on the average 160 pounds. Previous history, habits, and family history negative. His present illness began in October, 1913, with heavy burning pains in the epigastrium after eating. In November he noticed blood in the stools and occasionally vomited blood clots. He went to the hospital for two weeks, where he was partly on a bread and milk diet, and then stayed at home for eight weeks before going back to work. After four weeks the pain reappeared with the same symptoms. He was admitted to the University Hospital of Minnesota (Case No. 5356), on September 15, 1914. At this time the pain was absent, but an area of tenderness was noted over the stomach. He was thin, weak, unable to work, was constipated, with blood occasionally in the stools and blood clots occasionally in the vomitus. Physical examination showed him fairly well nourished, with marked anaemia, palpable cervical glands, submerged tonsils, had pyorrhoea and many old roots. The diagnosis was made as that of gastric ulcer, marked secondary anaemia, mitral insufficiency, apical abscesses and pyorrhoea. Hemoglobin 35%, red blood cells, 3,500,000, and leucocytes, 8,000.

Between September 15 and October 1 oral infection was eradicated. All remaining upper teeth were extracted, also the abscessed lower molars. The remaining lower teeth were treated for pyorrhoea.

On November 2 the physician in charge made the following note: "Patient's condition has remarkably improved. His weight has increased twenty-three pounds. There is no abdominal pain."

He was discharged on November 11, 1914, greatly improved, with no other treatment than a bread and milk diet and the elimination of the oral foci.

He again presented for examination in March, 1915. He had been working and living as a lumber man, eating a full mixed diet and doing the heaviest kind of work, and has been perfectly well since leaving the hospital. He states that for one and a half years before admission here, he had been troubled almost continuously with stomach symptoms and has never had so long a period of freedom as this before. A blood count at this time showed the hemoglobin to be 77%.

6. *Diseases of the Blood.*

Today we know that infections are never entirely localized. Bacteria, their toxins and protein poison, produced during the process of infection and inflammation, or both, are always absorbed into the circulation, not only from the primary focus, but also from secondary lesions.

The presence of bacteria and of protein poisons in the blood may cause diseases of violent and acute symptoms, or may be very latent in character, according to and depending on the number, virulence, and species of the bacteria, as well as the reaction and resisting quality of the defending blood cells.

SEPTICEMIA Septicemia is an acute general infection of the blood caused by bacteremia which occurs if living pyogenic bacteria exist and multiply in the blood.

Etiology: Septicemia often results from cases of extensive acute suppuration or from absorption of bacteria in open wounds. It is predisposed by high virulence of the bacteria and lowered resistance of the patient. It occurs especially after surgical interference in septic conditions in patients with lowered resistance, and from persistent toxic and bacterial absorption, as from acute abscesses without outlet from the pus. In patients who are feeble from a long standing infection it is therefore advisable not to remove all foci at once, or the result may be fatal. The streptococcus which is found in almost all oral infections is the cause of septicemia, but also other pyogenic bacteria may produce the disease.

Symptoms: After the inoculation the patient suffers from repeated chills, and the temperature rises to 105° F. The appetite is lost and the patient apathetic and delirious. The pulse becomes weaker and irregular and the temperature falls quickly before the exitus. Death usually occurs in a few days, but sometimes the end is drawn out for several weeks. The diagnosis of septicemia is made by the severe and rapid constitutional symptoms and is differentiated from toxemia and sapremia by the blood test. A blood culture should be made at once, using great care to disinfect the patient's skin. Blood is withdrawn from the median basillic vein by means of a sterile aspirating syringe, and cultures are made in the ordinary manner. If bacterial growth is obtained, we can make a sure diagnosis of septicemia.

Treatment: A great deal depends upon prompt, active and thorough treatment of the local lesion. A few hours make a great difference in the outcome. Free drainage should be established by a wide incision; hot, moist, and large dressings should be applied and changed every few minutes. Saline infusions (1000 to 3000 c.c.) are extremely useful; the diet should be regulated; and later, after the infection has subsided, tonics and stimulants should be given.

PYAEMIA Pyaemia is an acute infection of the blood characterized by the presence of infected emboli in the blood, which in turn cause metastatic abscesses wherever they lodge.

Etiology: The bacteria causing the infection in the primary focus produce coagulation of the blood. This clot soon becomes infected, and portions of it are broken off and thrown into the circulation. It follows the venous system, where it may cause thrombosis or be carried to the heart and be distributed into any part of the circulation. The streptococcus is the commonest cause of this disease, but like septicemia it may also be caused by the bacillus coli, staphylococcus, pneumococcus, and bacillus typhosus.

Symptoms: The symptoms are the same as of septicemia and usually start with a severe rigor followed by profuse sweating. The temperature is of intermittent character and rises up to 105° F. Abscesses usually make their appearance after a week and affect any part of the body. In chronic pyaemia the symptoms are less marked.

Treatment: The radical treatment of the primary focus is to be undertaken at once. The lesion should be freely opened, the septic material removed without disturbing the leucocytic area, which would allow absorption and further contaminate the blood stream. Establish free drainage and irrigate often. Anti-streptococcic serum may be used and also autogenous vaccine as soon as it can be made. The outcome of the disease depends upon the resistance of the patient and virulence of the bacteria and is often fatal.

ILLUSTRATIVE CASE *Case XVI.* (Pyemia.) (Reported by C. A. Haman, *Wisconsin Medical Journal,* March, 1903.) Patient, a man of forty years, seen in consultation with Dr. W. E. Bruner. An upper molar had been extracted a week preceding, the face was swollen from an alveolar abscess. The right eye was very prominent. He had a high evening temperature of 104 to 106° F., with morning intermissions. In a few days the other eye became prominent, which is quite ·characteristic of cavernous sinus thrombosis, and is accounted for by the venous connection between the teeth and periodontal structures and the cavernous sinus. The veins from the teeth empty into the pterygoid plexus. The pterygoid plexus communicates with the cavernous sinus directly by means of small veins passing through the foramen Vessalii, foramen orale and foramen lacerum medium, and indirectly through ·the facial vein which empties into the sinus. The diagnosis of sinus thrombosis was confirmed. The patient lived about a week.

TOXEMIA Toxemia is a term which expresses a condition due to the absorption of toxins. Toxin in its strictest meaning is produced only by a small number of bacteria, as we have already seen, such as the diphtheria and tetanus bacilli. Generally, however, we speak of toxemia as a condition which may be caused by the absorption of any poisonous substances originated from bacteria or bacterial activity. If the poison is produced by saprophytic bacteria which live on dead material, we speak of "sapremia."

Etiology: Toxemia is due to the absorption of poisons created by bacterial activity and tissue reaction. In true toxemia toxins only are absorbed from the focus, but the term is also applied to all those conditions where bacteria also have entered the circulation as long as these produce no acute general infection (septicemia).

Foci which cause toxemia are found in the intestinal tract, the genito-urinary system, and nose, and adjacent sinuses, the throat, and the oral cavity. Oral abscesses play the most important rôle in the mouth, but toxic absorption is also caused from unclean crown and bridge work, stomatitis, and pyorrhoea on account of the absorbing quality of the mucous membrane. All lesions in the mouth are caused or inhabited by the largest variety of pathogenic and saprophytic bacteria. They grow in combinations, inhabiting the diseased tissue simultaneously or acting at different stages of the decomposition, which makes possible the production of a large variety of chemical substances, as has already been described in the first part. These poisons may have special actions on certain tissues. It is well known that the diphtheria toxin, for example, is especially prone to attack the nervous system and to cause peripheral neuritis.

Symptoms: Toxemia may be very severe, beginning with chills, a rapid rise of temperature reaching 104° F.; there may be anorexia, headache and prostration, and later delirium, stupor or coma. In the less severe or chronic cases, which are of very frequent occurrence, the principal complaint is malaise.

MALAISE OR CHRONIC TOXEMIA Malaise is a condition caused by a certain amount of toxin or bacteria, or both, entering the circulation. The disease is not acute and violent as in acute septicemia and acute toxemia, probably on account of insufficient number and virility of the bacteria absorbed, and of the small amount of poison liberated to cause severe intoxication. The blood pressure is lowered and the symptoms are best expressed by the complaint of the patient of the inability of doing mentally or physically the accustomed day's work. Slight exertions cause disproportionate fatigue. An abnormal amount of rest is required, the appetite is often poor, the skin has usually a grayish, sallow appearance, the lips lack the color of health, there is loss of weight, constipation, and benumbed mental activity.

Treatment: The foci may not be apparent, and it may require a thorough search to locate the lesion from which the absorption takes place. It should be remembered that a very small focus may, on account of its persistence and its chronic nature, cause a small but continuous infection of the blood. The radical removal of such foci is the first step in the treatment; there is frequently more than one focus and it is important to remove all the septic conditions. If the tonsils are diseased, it does not mean that oral abscesses may not participate. The treatment of the cause is often sufficient to result in a cure; in other cases, it is advisable to give tonics and stimulants.

ILLUSTRATIVE CASES *Case XVII.* (Toxemia.) Patient, a young lady, a college student, consulted me about a tooth which had been unsuccessfully treated. She had no symptoms of discomfort in her mouth, but upon questioning, complained of a tired feeling and frequent intermittent fever of about eight months standing. A radiograph showed a lower six-year molar with poor root-canal filling, but no pronounced periapical destruction. The second bicuspid, which is the tooth in question, presented a very large area of lessened density at the distal side of the apex. The tooth was at once extracted and the bone curetted. The patient improved rapidly; the fever did not recur. (Figure 156.)

Case XVIII. (Toxemia.) Patient, a man of middle age, asked two years ago for a careful examination of his teeth. He complained of an intoxicated feeling in his head, which manifested itself principally in the morning. His ability to think was greatly decreased, smoking made him ill, while before he was able to smoke a moderate amount. Radiographs of his teeth showed abscesses on the upper right incisor, upper left cuspid, first and second bicuspid. I opened these teeth; a vile odor came from the canals. Apiectomy was performed on the lateral incisor after the root canal was properly treated and filled. The cuspid and two bicuspids I cleaned thoroughly with the sulphuric acid method, and treated the canals with formocresol, and ionic medication. The root canals were filled, but the points projected through the apical foramen. During the treatment the patient improved greatly and at the end his head felt perfectly clear so that he could again do his ordinary day's work. He also said that he was again able to smoke without discomfort. After eight months he came back saying that the old trouble recurred in a mild form. A new radiograph showed the areas of lessened density the same as before the treatment. I amputated the roots of the two bicuspids at once, and later I performed the same operation on the cuspid. The patient reported an almost immediate change, and so far, permanent improvement. He later told me of another condition which apparently came from the teeth. He had the upper bicuspid tooth treated in Paris some time preceding and remembered distinctly that from this date he was afflicted with constipation. After the first treatment of the teeth he got rid of this condition entirely, and did not need any drugs until it returned with the toxemia. Again it was permanently relieved after the surgical removal of the abscesses. The interesting part about this case is the fact proven that root canal treatment neither with antiseptic nor ionic medication cured the abscess permanently, although the treatment was thorough and much longer continued than was necessary according to general rules. The bacterial growth and production of toxin was inhibited for a few months, but was only lying dormant until the infectious process slowly recovered. (Figures 157, 158.)

ANAEMIA Anaemia is a reduction in the amount of blood as a whole or of its corpuscles, or of certain of its constituents. There is primary or idiopathic anaemia due to increased destruction due to some existing disease. Among the primary anaemias belong chlorosis, a disease of young girls, and pernicious anaemia, the cause of which is not definitely understood. Among the secondary anaemias belong acute and chronic secondary anaemia. Hunter separates a special class which he calls septic anaemia.

PERNICIOUS ANAEMIA Pernicious anaemia, or Addison's anaemia, Hunter says, is characterized by imperfect action of the blood-making organs, the absence of haemalytic and bone marrow changes, and characterized by pigment changes in the liver, kidney, and spleen. The disease is usually fatal.

Hunter, who has done so much good work on this subject, thinks that a large number of cases grouped as pernicious anaemia are really of an infectious nature with no bone marrow and pigment changes. The true pernicious anaemia, however, he regards as a chronic infective disease in which gastric disturbances, altered digestion, absorption and auto-intoxication, as well as oral abscesses and pyorrhoea alveolaris, may be a most important antecedent and concomitant, but not the only etiological factors. They precede the disease-creating conditions which permit the contraction of the specific (haemalytic) infection underlying the real characteristic features of the disease.

SEPTIC ANAEMIA Septic anaemia is a term used by Hunter for all cases of secondary anaemia which are of a septic infectious nature. Many of the cases diagnosed as pernicious anaemia, and especially all anaemias comprised within Biermer's definition of progressive pernicious anaemia, show a predominant septic factor. These are distinguished from pernicious or Addison's anaemia by the absence of haemalytic and bone marrow changes and absence of pigment changes in kidneys, liver, and spleen.

Etiology: Septic anaemia is caused by absorption of bacteria or the poisons of bacterial activity and may come from foci in the nose, sinuses of the oral cavity (abscesses, pyorrhoea), and infections in the stomach and intestine, or chronic suppuration in any other part of the body. Prognosis is favorable if the cause is removed in time, but the disease may have a severe and fatal course.

Symptoms: Dirty yellow, anaemic complexion, loss of bodily and mental vigor, with loss of weight. Not infrequently there is slight fever. The red blood corpuscles are reduced, but seldom below two millions, and haemoglobin is about forty-five per cent. on the average.

ILLUSTRATIVE CASE *Case XIX.* (Anaemia.) (Reported by T. B. Hartzel, *Journal of the Allied Dental Societies,* October, 1914, page 52.) This is one case out of four which came under the observation of the writer. The patient, a Scandinavian of fifty-three years, presented himself with a history of his illness, having started seven years ago with slight at-

PLATE XLVII

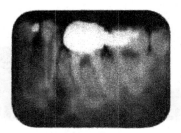

Fig. 156

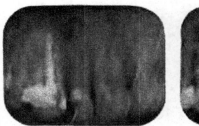

Fig. 157

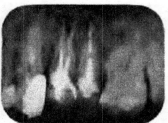

Fig. 158

Fig. 156.—Radiograph showing right lower second bicuspid causing toxemia in Case No. 17.

Figs. 157 and 158.—Radiographs of Case No. 18, showing four granulomata.

PLATE XLVIII

FIG. 159

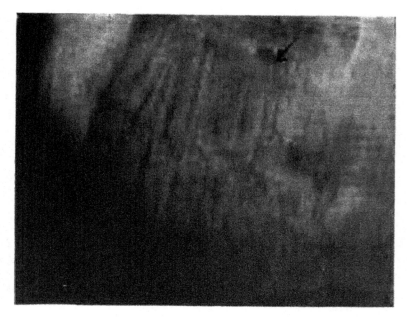

FIG. 159a

FIGS. 159 and 159a.—Radiographic plates of Case No. 20. The arrows indicate the granulomata.

tacks for a few minutes each day of chills and fever, followed by vomiting. These attacks had no relation to his meals. Since this time he had gradually, but intermittently, grown weaker. He had trouble for some time with swelling of the limbs and with dizziness. His color became pale and yellow, and he grew dull and listless. When admitted to the Eliott Hospital in Minneapolis, Minnesota, he was weak, yellow in color, with constant pain in his stomach, and seemed only dully conscious. The case was diagnosed by the medical staff as pernicious anaemia, with slight cardiac enlargement, mild pyorrhoea alveolaris and rarefaction about two root ends. He was put on iron and arsenites, and there seemed to be but little improvement, except a slight improvement in the blood count, until his mouth was put in good condition by the dental staff. Since that time he has been steadily improving. His consciousness had returned to normal and his other symptoms have been much improved. The most striking picture, however, is presented by his blood count, which has steadily risen from 900,000 red blood corpuscles and 15% haemoglobin to 2,630,000 red blood corpuscles and 61% haemoglobin. The only serious setback occurred June 16, which was coincident with the occurrence of a dental abscess, at which time the haemoglobin dropped back from 61% to 55%, and the red blood cells from 2,630,000 to 1,800,000. After extraction of the abscessed tooth, the last blood count jumped from 1,800,000 to 2,500,000, and the haemoglobin is the highest it has been since commencing his record, namely, 65%.

7. Diseases of the Heart.

The infective diseases of the heart are caused by haematogenous infection due frequently to the streptococcus viridans, but may also occur in connection with typhoid fever, pneumonia, influenza, diphtheria, tuberculosis, and syphilis. Dr. Richard C. Cabot, in an analysis of six hundred successive and unselected cases of heart disease, found that he could group 93% of these six hundred cases under four etiological headings: 1, Rheumatic, that is, presumably streptococci, 46%; 2, Nephritic, 19%; 3, Arteriosclerotic, 15%, and 4, Syphilitic, 12%. The streptococcic infections of the heart have their origin in a large majority of cases before the twenty-second year. It begins young, it is essentially a chronic disease, and if severe or progressive, handicaps those afflicted during the prime of life, and often causes death before maturity. On account of the severe prognosis, every effort should be made to eliminate all septic foci in the body as a preventive measure, especially the ones which are liable to be caused and harbor the streptococcus. Streptococcic infections of the tonsils and teeth are of very frequent occurrence in children and form an ideal entrance for disease. At this place it is necessary again to call attention to the importance of removing both tonsilar and dental foci, both on account of the intimate relation between these organs and the danger of the persistence from a seemingly unimportant lesion after the principal ones have been removed. The temporary teeth, especially the temporary molars, are very often pulpless and abscessed and suffered to remain in the mouth, partly because they cause no pain and partly for orthodontic reasons. It is, however, much better to sacrifice those temporary teeth and take a chance on the possibility of malocclusion rather than on the possibility of heart infection and life itself.

The pericardium, myocardium, and the valves, have the same general blood supply and therefore they are all liable to haematogenous infection resulting in pericarditis, myocarditis, and endocarditis (valvular and mural).

PERICARDITIS Pericarditis is an infection of the pericardium occurring in children at an early age. Its most frequent etiological factor is systemic infection from infections in other parts of the body, but it also may occur as a continuous infection from diseases of the pleura as well as the myocardium.

MYOCARDITIS The cardiac musculature very frequently becomes attacked by secondary infections; it may be due to the streptococcus, the gonococcus, the pneumococcus, or other microörganisms. The microscope reveals lesions in the heart muscle which explain cardiac irritability and later indications of cardiac distress from infective diseases.

ENDOCARDITIS Endocarditis is the inflammation of the lining membrane of the heart, and is usually confined to the valves (valvular endocarditis) and rarely to the walls (mural endocarditis). It is principally caused by the streptococcus and especially by the streptococcus viridans (rheumatism), which may be transported from a primary focus, such as the tonsils, abscesses on the teeth, etc. The streptococcus causing endocarditis grows best in high oxygen tension, and is usually extremely virulent. The circulating blood furnishes oxygen in abundance and furnishes an ideal condition for an abundant vegetative growth on the valves and walls of the endocardium. Syphilis, that is, the spirochaeta pallida, is another important etiological factor. Typhoid, scarlet fever, pneumonia, influenza, diphtheria, and tuberculosis occasionally involve the valves, but show a marked predilection for the myocardium.

Endocarditis occurs in two forms: acute endocarditis, characterized by the presence of vegetation with loss of continuity (simple endocarditis), or of substance in the valve tissues (ulcerative endocarditis); chronic endocarditis is a slow sclerotic change, resulting in thickening and deformity.

Treatment: The infectious diseases of the heart are of a very grave and often fatal nature. Careful study leads specialists to believe that in a large number of instances heart disease in the adult originates in childhood, and all energies should be put into the recognition and treatment of these diseases in the early stages. Eustis* says that endocarditis in its earliest stages is not surely recogni-

* Endocarditis in Children. *Boston Medical and Surgical Journal*, September 2, 1915.

zable, but that it is important to begin treatment, in order to be effective, before a diagnosis can be made. This means that infectious diseases as rheumatic (the term used in its broadest sense) attacks, and chorea in children should be treated as cases of acute endocarditis. In these cases of suspicious heart disease, we should remove septic foci, such as diseased tonsils or abscessed teeth. It should be remembered that absence of pain in the mouth or teeth is not a sign of healthy condition, but on the contrary, that the most dangerous septic foci, chronic abscesses, are often entirely symptomless and unsuspected by the patient, and that sometimes, if the removal of diseased tonsils does not give the desired result, there may be an unknown focus on one or more teeth which can only be discovered by the radiograph. Such a focus, although small, may be the cause of persistent infection. In removing such foci it is of greatest importance not to go about it in a wholesale manner; this might result in absolute harm. Eustis reports a heart case where a severe relapse of chorea occurred immediately after the extraction of several teeth. The practice of removing tonsils, adenoids, and abscessed teeth, all at one time, is very frequently undertaken in order to save the patient repeated shocks of general anaesthesia, but is poor policy, as it is liable to cause exacerbations of the disease we try to cure. The foci should be removed gradually, the tonsils separately, and the teeth one by one; this can be done easily and without causing great shock if local anaesthesia is used, which is a most excellent method for operations in the mouth. It also gives the operator a much better chance to curette and inspect the abscess cavity, a most important part of the operation.

The recovery from heart diseases is extremely slow; strict rest in bed for weeks or months is almost universally advised in these cases even for several weeks after the temperature and pulse have reached normal. This is a most difficult thing I find for many dentists to understand; they think the patient should recover immediately after the foci in the mouth have been removed.

ILLUSTRATIVE CASE *Case XX.* (Subacute endocarditis.) The patient, a boy, aged thirteen, born in Russia. He had been in this country for two years. He had had the measles when very young and scarlet fever some five years before coming to this country. He never had had any sore throat.

Seven months ago he started to have pain in the joints, mostly in the shoulder region, associated with fever. Shortly afterwards he complained of pain over the precardia and of dyspnea upon exertion. He was kept in bed except for meals.

Physical examination showed lungs negative; heart, apex visible and palpable in fifth interspace, 11 c.m. from the midsternum. Over the apex was felt a distinct presystolic thrill. Sounds of a fair quality but rapid. At mitral area is heard a presystolic murmur. Over aorta is a diastolic murmur and over pulmonic area is a systolic murmur. Abdomen is full, soft, and tympanitic throughout. No masses or tenderness. Knee jerks present. No glands in neck, axilla, or groin. Pulse equal, regular, of waterhammer variety. Capillary pulse present.

Patient was admitted to the Robert B. Brigham hospital on November 6. Temperature 100.6° F.; pulse, 140; respiration, 28; blood pressure, 125-80. He was put on a light diet and kept in bed. I ordered X-rays taken of his teeth, which showed shadows representing granulomata at the roots of the two lower first molars and one upper first molar. I extracted the upper first molar on December 11, and the right lower first molar on December 14, both under local anaesthesia. Cultures from the upper molar revealed a streptococcus and staphylococcus infection. From the lower molar a pure streptococcus infection was demonstrated. On December 23 a slight downward tendency of temperature was reported, the pulse still being variable. He received vaccine treatment beginning January 10, 1915, which, however, did not improve his condition. On February 3, the third six-year molar was extracted, and yielded a streptococcus culture.

The patient improved materially after this and was advised to have his tonsils out, as they were enlarged, but left the hospital on February 28 at his father's request. He was again examined at the hospital in *June*, 1916. He was greatly improved: no temperature, better pulse, is able to go about and to attend school.   Regurgitation and mitral stenosis are still present and will probably remain as permanent defects.   (Figure 159.)

8. *Affections of the Nervous System.*

Nerve affections due to oral conditions are either local, remote, or general. The local conditions arise from direct infection of the branches of the maxillary or mandibular division of the fifth nerve by septic condition, or are caused by pressure, such as is frequently caused by impacted and unerupted teeth.   The pain is usually referred to other branches of the fifth or to communicating nerves which may result in complaints in other organs such as the ear and eye, where not infrequently aural or ophthalmic disturbances are produced by the referred irritation.   These conditions have already been described under their respective headings. If nerves in other parts of the body are infected, we speak of remote infection, and if a large number is involved, we speak of general nerve infection. The two latter conditions are caused by haematogenous infection or intoxication. The bacteria and poisons created by bacterial activity or the latter alone are absorbed from the primary focus and certain toxins are thought to have a special affinity for the nervous system. The poisoned blood irritates the nerves and causes certain disturbances such as neuritis, chorea, insomnia, and mental depression.

NEURITIS   Neuritis is an inflammation of the nerve trunks; it may be in a single nerve localized, "or involving a large number of nerves," called general or multiple neuritis.

Etiology: Localized neuritis is usually caused by cold, traumatism, or extension of inflammation from neighboring parts. This condition is of frequent occurrence in the mouth. Alveolar abscesses, or impacted teeth, maxillary sinusitis, and osteomyelitis often involve inflammation of parts of the second or third division of the fifth nerve. Postoperative pains after operations on the jaws are also well known and are due to traumatic injury of or continuous traumatic inflammation of the nerves.

General neuritis has a very complex etiology: organic poisons, as alcohol, ether, lead, arsenic, mercury, etc., and poisons caused by infections, such as streptococcus, infections, diphtheria, typhoid fever, smallpox, scarlet fever, syphilis, and others.

Hunter and other authors think that oral sepsis plays a great rôle in the etiology of toxin neuritis. Hunter* gives three well-studied cases of typical general neuritis prevailing for many years (Case 3 for fourteen years), and in all cases there resulted immediate improvement from the removal of the septic oral conditions.

Symptoms: In localizing neuritis there is pain of a boring or stabbing character felt in the course of the nerve and in the parts supplied. In general neuritis there is no constant intense pain in the nerves, but there is numbness and tingling in the hands and arms or part supplied, a so-called paresthesia, which is often described as the "pins and needles" sensation. There may also be alterations in the muscular power and abolition of deep reflexes.

ILLUSTRATIVE CASE *Case XXI.* (Local neuritis.) The patient, a woman of about thirty-seven years, complained of local neuritis in the lower jaw. An X-ray plate was taken and showed a large area of lessened density about a root in the lower jaw. The inflammatory process involved in this case the inferior alveolar nerve and was the direct cause of the neuritis. After removal of the root and curettage, followed by occasional treatment, the condition disappeared completely. (Figure 160.)

---

* HUNTER: Pernicious anæmia, pp. 303-305.

TRIFACIAL NEURALGIA Neuralgia is a pain in a nerve or nerves of radiating character. Trigeminal neuralgia attacks mostly only one branch of the nerve, but in rarer cases two or all divisions may be involved. It is characteristic for the disease that no inflammatory conditions occur in the part where the pain is located.

Etiology: The cause of trigeminal neuralgia is frequently of obscure character and often cannot be located even after the most painstaking search. It is said to occur from general and local causes. The general causes are a result of toxemia such as produced by infectious diseases. The local causes are more important. They may be due to diseases of the eye, middle ear, nose and accessory sinuses, or especially the oral cavity and teeth.

The diseases of the oral cavity most commonly cause trifacial neuralgia. Pulpstones or nodules often occur in the pulp chamber of a tooth, causing pressure upon the nerve fibres of the pulp. Impacted and unerupted teeth are also an important factor. The pressure exerted by a developing tooth which grows in a wrong direction may be extremely great and sometimes even causes absorption of parts of the permanent tooth which stands in its way, even exposing its nerve. Pieces of alveolar process are sometimes fractured after extraction and escape discovery, or such pieces or ends of roots may be forced into the cancellous part of the bone and cause, especially in the lower jaw on account of the mandibular canal, pressure upon the nerve. Abscesses on unerupted and impacted teeth and chronic abscesses in general may, besides being a focus from which toxic absorption takes place, be the cause of trigeminal neuralgia. They usually give no local discomfort, but may be causing irritation and inflammation of branches of the fifth nerve, causing in turn a reflex neuralgic condition.

Symptoms: The pain many times is only a slight and bearable one, but in other cases it is of most excruciating character. Some patients have a continuous mild pain with severe attacks at irregular intervals. The interim,

PLATE XLIX

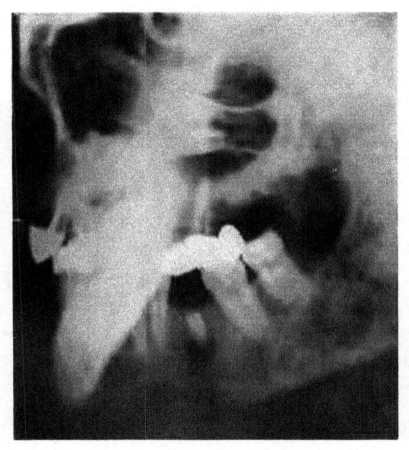

FIG. 160

FIG. 160.—Radiographic plate of Case No. 21, showing a large osteo-myelitic area caused by the root which remained under a bridge. The diseased area extends into the mandibular canal causing neuritis of the inferior alveolar nerve.

PLATE L

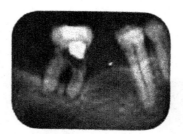

FIG. 161

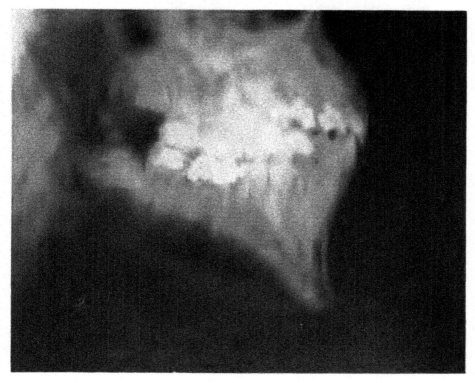

FIG. 162

FIG. 161.—Radiograph of lower molar with cavity beneath the gum (dark area around the filling) of Case No. 22.

FIG. 162.—Radiographic plate showing impacted lower third molar which caused neuralgia in Case No. 23.

during which the patient is either free of pain or where there is only a dull aching, may last minutes, hours, or days. The attacks sometimes are of such terrible character that the patient is tempted to commit suicide.

The attacks occur either spontaneously or may be induced by movements of the mouth, washing of the face, or touching the lips or cheek with the fingers.

Diagnosis: Diagnosis of trigeminal neuralgia requires the most painstaking search for general as well as local causes. It is principally a process of elimination of one possible cause after the other. The use of the radiograph is imminent for examination of the oral cavity. Plates should be taken first to make sure that there are no impacted, unerupted, or supernumerary teeth or odontomas in remote parts of the maxillary or mandibular bones. The plates also give us a general idea about the teeth. Films from different angles should then be taken of all the teeth for a more detailed diagnosis, and only the very best negatives are good enough to ascertain the presence or absence of abscesses and pulpstones.

Dr. Henry Head believes that neuralgic pains resulting from teeth have definite areas of reference in relation to the tooth involved. These areas have been ascertained by gently pinching the loose skin, and if the right spot is touched, there is often a distinct exacerbation of pain from the tooth. The following table is from Behan's book on "Pain."

Tooth	Reference Area	
Maxill. Incisors	Fronto nasal region	
Maxill. Cuspid	Naso labial region	
Maxill. First Bicuspid	Naso labial region	
Maxill. Second Bicuspid	Temp'l or maxillary	
Maxill. First Molar	Maxillary region	
Maxill. Second Molar	Mandibular region	
Maxill. Third Molar	Mandibular region	
Mand. Incisors	Mental region	
Mand. Cuspid	Mental region	
Mand. First Bicuspid	Mental region	
Mand. Second Bicuspid	Hyoid or mental	
Mand. First Molar	Hyoid	Also in ear and just behind
Mand. Second Molar	Hyoid	angle of jaw and tip of
Mand. Third Molar	Sup. Laryngeal	tongue on same side.

Treatment: Treatment of neuralgia consists of removal of the cause and treatment of the symptoms. In cases of obscure persistent nature, alcohol injection into the main trunks or the Gasserian ganglion are recommended. Neurectomy of the terminal branches or of the whole second or third division is advocated by the believers in the surgical methods, and as a last resort the removal of the Gasserian ganglion.

ILLUSTRATIVE CASES
Case XXII. (Trifacial neuralgia.) Patient, Mrs. S., was referred to me for radiographic examination to find the cause of an obscure neuralgia, which was referred to the right upper side of the jaws. A diseased condition of the bone in the upper jaw was suspected by her dentist. The radiograph, however, revealed an obscure pus condition about the root of the lower second molar concealed by the gum, causing necrosis of the root. The extraction of the lower molar stopped the neuralgia entirely. (Figure 161.)

Case XXIII. (Trifacial neuralgia.) Patient, a young lady, complained of faceaches on the left side, which sometimes were very severe and interfered with her studies. X-ray showed an impacted lower wisdom tooth as well as abscesses on both ends of the first molar. I extirpated the impacted tooth, extracted the first molar, and curetted the abscess cavities. The patient made quick recovery and has been free of pain ever since. (Figure 162.)

CHOREA
Chorea, or St. Vitus's Dance, is a disease chiefly affecting children, characterized by irregular, involuntary contraction of the muscles, and a marked association with acute endocarditis and rheumatism.

Etiology: The disease is most common in children between the age of five and fifteen. Fright, injury, and mental worry are named as etiological factors; the principal cause, however, seems to be of an infectious nature. It has already been said that chorea is closely related to endocarditis and rheumatism, which diseases we know to be due to streptococcemia, thanks to our modern understanding enlightened by the splendid work of Rosenow.

The foci which are looked for in the streptococcus infections (arthritis, endocarditis) are therefore also possible foci for chorea, and practical experience confirms this supposition. Eustis* mentions two relapses, one of arthritis and one of chorea following tonsilectomy, and also reports another case where a severe relapse of chorea followed immediately after the extraction of several teeth. These relapses are due to an increased amount of bacteria absorbed from the unprotected wound and again teaches us to remove such foci one by one with an interval of several days between each extraction or operation.

ILLUSTRATIVE CASE *Case XXIV.* (Chorea.) (Reported by M. T. Schamberg, *Journal of the Allied Dental Societies,* December, 1915.) A young girl, about fifteen years of age, was sent to the hospital with the following complications of diseases: chorea, muscular rheumatism, and a valvular lesion of the heart. She was observed in the medical ward and treated for some time without material improvement. When she was finally sent to Dr. Schamberg's clinic, the jactitation and convulsive movements of her body almost interfered with a thorough examination of her mouth. Yet, staring us in the face was a gold crown upon an upper front tooth. An X-ray was made of this part and an infection detected. The removal of the tooth and curettage of the bone was promptly followed by an improvement in the chorea, and at the end of several weeks the patient walked with scarcely any evidence of the disease. There was likewise such a pronounced improvement in her other conditions that she was considered well enough to be dismissed from the hospital.

MELANCHOLIA AND MENTAL DEPRESSION Mental depression and melancholia are diseases or perhaps symptoms of a more or less obscure nature. While it seems a far cry from oral infections to mental diseases, we have reliable reports from sincere men who have seen profound depression and melancholy disappear

---

* EUSTIS: Endocarditis in Children. *Boston Medical and Surgical Journal,* September 2, 1915.

after the treatment or surgical removal of septic foci in the mouth. Such cures are convincing arguments that chronic intoxications from septic foci are some of the etiological factors in these conditions.

ILLUSTRATIVE CASE *Case XXV.* (Mental depression with oral sepsis as an important factor.) (Reported by C. Burns Graig.) The patient a woman aged fifty-nine, well preserved, and of more than average mentality. She came from a long-lived, non-nervous stock. The father died three years ago, the mother two years ago. During the week of the mother's death she had a nasal operation. Soon after this, financial losses caused considerable worry. The patient continued in reasonably good health for over a year. At this time she went to a fashionable sanitarium, more as a pleasure resort than for treatment. While there, she began to have attacks of dizziness. A physician told her she had mild heart disease and prescribed Nauheim baths. After she had taken eleven baths a nervous breakdown began.

When first seen, the patient was greatly depressed and nearly always in a state of agitation, at other times she spoke in a mournful tone without being able to give the exact cause of her depression. She said she was convinced she would not recover.

Physical examination was entirely negative except pulse of 100 and condition of her teeth. Radiograms showed two abscesses on the roots of crowned teeth and a collection of pus beneath a faulty bridge. The stools when examined proved normal, except slight evidence of catarrhal colitis. Haemoglobin, 78%. Red blood cells, 4,869,000. White blood cells, 6,500; differential showed mild increase in the lymphocytes. Urine normal. A test breakfast showed diminution in the hydrochloric acid content. A serum Wasserman was negative and the spinal fluid was normal in every respect.

A week of tonic measures was without noticeable improvement. It was then decided to have the bridge work removed and the abscesses cured. During the following week the cloud began to lift and the patient began to have moments of better humor, and saw some possibility of looking at the brighter side of things. She was then sent to the country for two weeks from whence she returned in a comparatively happy state of mind.

Case XXVI. (Melancholia.) (Reported by Van Doorn, *Dental Cosmos,* June, 1909.) The patient, a young lady, was referred to Dr. Van Doorn as a case of melancholia. The patient had as little cause for mental depression as one could possibly imagine, of which she was as well aware as the doctor. She had wealth, friends, a beautiful home, and the education and culture that should go with such a happy environment. Examination of the mouth revealed nothing serious. Radiographs taken by Dr. Lodge revealed a number of teeth with areas of absorption about their apices, of the existence of which she had not the slightest idea. Some of the teeth were extracted, others could be saved by treatment. Within a short time after the septic foci in the mouth had been removed, the patient was in normal condition. She had no recurrence of her melancholia up to the time of the essay (about one year).

9. *Diseases of the Joints.*

ACUTE INFECTIOUS ARTHRITIS Acute infectious arthritis, or rheumatic fever, is an acute infection of the joints to focal disease. In children, carditis and chorea often occur simultaneously; in adults, the systemic infection involves the heart less frequently.

The disease usually starts with irregular pains in the joints and slight malaise. There is slight chilliness, the fever rises quickly and within twenty-four hours the disease is fully manifest. Temperature between 102 and 104° F. Pulse soft and usually above 100. The affected joints are painful to move, soon become swollen and hot and present a reddish flush. The disease is seldom limited to a single articulation and the joints are usually attacked successively. The course of the disease is extremely variable and depends whether there are also cardiac (endocarditis, myocarditis, pericarditis), pulmonary (pneumonia and pleurisy), and nervous (chorea, meningitis, polyneuritis, coma) affections.

Etiology: The newer methods of bacterial culture (Rosenow) have proved the presence of infectious organisms in the joint fluid, in the synovial membrane and proximal lymphnodes where it may always be found during the height of the disease. The organisms belong to the diplococcus, streptococcus class. The focus is principally found in the throat (tonsils), nose, and accessory sinuses, and the oral cavity.

Case XXVII. (Acute Infectious Arthritis.) Patient, a man, about thirty-four years of age, was sent to me for treatment. Had had measles followed by mumps, but no other childhood diseases. A month before consulting me he had rheumatic swellings and pain in the knees. The shoulders were next attacked, and after a short time all the large joints became involved. He took electric baths but did not improve.

He was able to walk only with crutches. He showed me radiographs which had been taken of his teeth. There were areas of lessened density on the right upper central incisor and the left upper first molar. The broach which the dentist had inserted into the root canal extended directly into the antrum and a frontal plate of both antra showed an opaque area on the left side. I operated, opening through the canine fossa; there was a large abscess at the floor of the antrum. I extracted the troublesome molar and removed by curettage the diseased bone and abscessed areas. The antrum was washed daily. Apiectomy was then performed on the central incisor.

The patient suffered an exacerbation in the knee joint and had to stay in bed for three days. After a week he started to improve gradually and after seven weeks, when the antrum had healed, he was entirely rid of arthritis. He walked into my office without difficulty; his joints were

PLATE LI

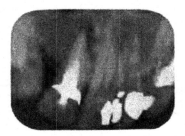

FIG. 163

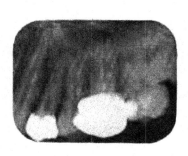

FIG. 164

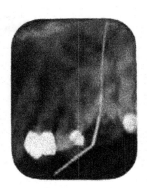

FIG. 165

FIGS. 163, 164 and 165.—Radiographs of Case No. 27. There is an abscess on the upper central incisor and upper first molar, which infected the antrum causing acute arthritis of all the joints.

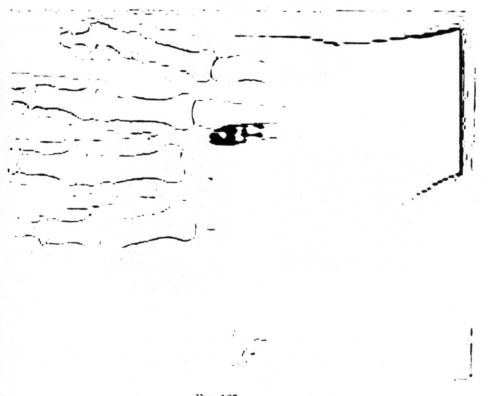

Fig. 167

Fig. 166.—Normal hand.

Hypertrophic Arthritis.   Note the boty overgrowth of many of the phalangeal joints,
especially the terminal of the first and fifth phalanges.

normal. He received no general treatment while I took care of him, and the improvement in the condition of the joints was wholly due to the removal of the infectious focus. (Figures 163 to 165.)

HYPERTRO-PHIC ARTHRITIS Hypertrophic arthritis is the term used by Goldthwaite, Painter, and Osgood for those cases in which the chief lesion is an outgrowth of bone in or very near the joint, but without destruction of joint tissue as a characteristic or important change. Most writers agree to classify these cases as hypertrophic, except Billings, who would deny this condition a class by itself, placing it in the group with atrophic arthritis as a result of joint infection. (Figure 167.)

It is a disease of the latter half of life. There is usually a history of trauma, or static disturbances. The disease does not show a tendency to steady progression. There is no true ankylosis, motion is limited only by interference of the exostoses. The X-ray shows the presence of osteophytic outgrowths and marked marginal lipping of the joints.

Etiology: Painter, who also recognizes the type of hypertrophic arthritis, believes it is not due to infection, but to a combination of trauma and faulty metabolism.

GOUTY ARTHRITIS Gouty arthritis should not be confused with true gout, for many of the characteristics are lacking. It is a disease of the metabolism which may attack any damaged joint. It derives its name from the fact that the bones show the small pouched out spots called "Bruce's nodes," which are also found in true gout. (Figure 168.)

CHRONIC IN-FECTIOUS AND ATROPHIC ARTHRITIS Painter divides the chronic infectious type of arthritis into infectious and atrophic. It has been established that the infectious group is found in earlier life, while the atrophic type is seen in persons of older age. In the Robert B. Brigham Hospital Painter classified twenty-five cases and showed that the average age of the infectious type is thirty-two years, of the atrophic type forty-nine years. "It seems, therefore, logical to suppose," says Lawrence, "that atrophic and infectious arthritis are but different stages of the same process." The chronic infectious type, which occurs in early life, is called Still's disease in children.

Etiology: Chronic infections and their sequel, atrophic arthritis, are much more common and more serious than the hypertrophic form. The two main causes of these two types are now generally held to be autointoxication and infection. (Figures 169 and 170.)

Autointoxication is by some writers believed the etiological factor, because many investigators (Phillip, Cole, Beattie, and others) failed entirely to demonstrate bacteria in the diseased joints. The toxin material may come from any part of the body and may be due either to continuous, persistent bacterial activity in some focus discharging toxins into the blood (toxemia), or to metabolic or digestive derangements.

Bacterial infection of the joint tissue is believed to be the cause by other writers, Schüller, Poynton, Paine, and before all, Rosenow isolated three organisms belonging to the streptococcus pneumococcus group from the joints. Each of these organisms is convertible into the other types by cultural methods. These bacteria have a characteristic low grade virulence and grow best in a low oxygen tension and even grow anaerobically. Such a condition is found in the infected joints caused by the method by which the bacteria invade the tissue; the vessels supplying the joints are closed by endothelial proliferation at the site and stimulated by the bacterial embolus. Injected into animals they produce arthritis, endocarditis, pericarditis, myositis, and myocarditis. Steinharter* undertook such animal experiments, injecting staphylococcus cultures into rabbits and dogs intravenously. The material used was prepared by suspending an agar slant culture in about 10 c.c. of normal salt solution. The usual dose of such an emulsion was 1 c.c. for a rabbit and 3 c.c. for a dog. The results as shown by the published protocols, indicate that the staphylococcus is apt to localize in the joints and pro-

---

* *See* Bibliography.

PLATE LIII

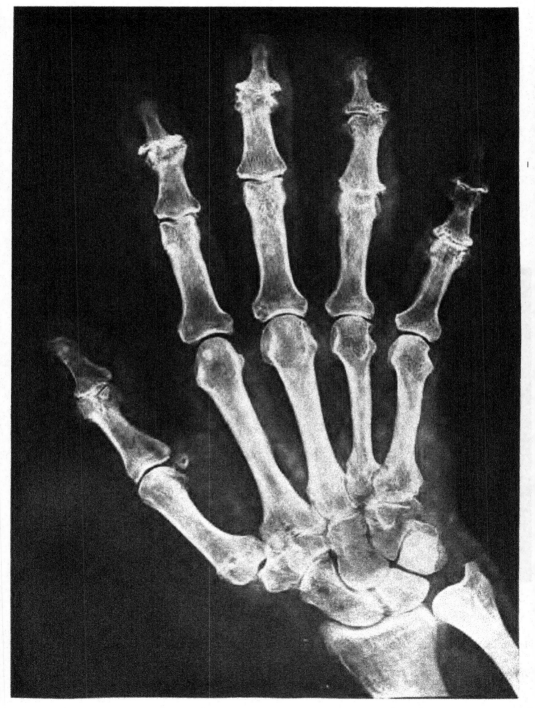

FIG. 168.—Gouty Arthritis. Note hypertrophic changes of the phalangeal joints and the small areas having a pouched out appearance just posterior to the distal end of the second portion of the phalanges, characteristic of gout.

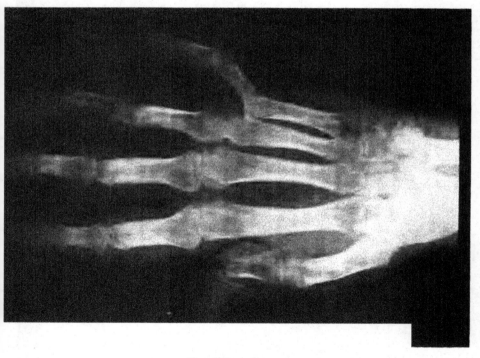

FIG. 170

Infectious Arthritis. Note the periarticular swelling and irregular joint atrophy with thinning of the cartilage.

Atrophic Arthritis. Note the general bony atrophic destruction of several joints with corresponding deformity.

duce the typical lesions and symptoms (lameness) of arthritis. The organisms recovered from the arthritic lesions have a decided tendency to again localize in joints. In some cases the arthritis was the only lesion found at autopsy, but in other cases it was associated with duodenal ulcer, appendicitis, cholecystitis, myocarditis, pericarditis, endocarditis, nephritis, colitis, and myositis. "The results of localization obtained in connection with studies of staphylococci," says the writer, "are singularly suggestive of Rosenow's results with streptococci."

The causative focus, is, according to Billings, usually found in the head, but may be found anywhere in the body. The most important places for infectious foci are found in the nose, throat (tonsils), oral cavity, the intestinal tract, and genito-urinary system. Septic foci may occur in different parts of the body simultaneously, as the tonsils and the teeth, or the teeth and the intestinal tract, and even may have a pathological connection. It is rather seldom to find a true condition where, for example, the only foci are found in the mouth, but it is evident that the sufferers from chronic arthritis have almost always an abundant number of septic lesions in the mouth, which without question may have been responsible for the disease. The lesions in the mouth from which haematogenous infection may take place are principally the different varieties of abscesses, pyorrhoea pockets, and septic bridgework. The streptococcus is most frequently found in oral abscesses, as has already been mentioned, and septic processes are found in the mouth of a very large percentage of people. At the Robert B. Brigham Hospital I examined eighty-seven patients, from which number seventy-two or eighty-nine per cent. had abscesses on from one to thirty-two teeth. The seventy-two patients had three hundred and forty abscesses and many suffered from pyorrhoea besides.

Treatment: The treatment consists in general improvement of the metabolism by suitable diet and open-air existence. Then comes the search and removal of all possible foci of infection and absorption to eliminate radically any source which was originally responsible for the disease and may cause reinfection. The removal of the focus does not necessarily result in a cure, as the secondary joint lesions have developed to a certain extent, but it frees the system from the burden of continuously taking care of those conditions and gives the patient a chance for an effort towards recovery from other diseased conditions. Abscesses, as well as other pus conditions in the mouth, should therefore be radically removed, not only because the system absorbs from them bacteria and toxins, but also because many have sinuses into the mouth through which pus is discharged, which deteriorate the food and cause gastric and intestinal sepsis. It is also important to restore the masticatory apparatus to full efficiency. The teeth, which are missing, should be replaced by plates or by removable bridge work, because it is not fair to expect that the stomach of a weakened patient will digest food which has not been properly prepared in the mouth. Local treatment of the diseased joints and consists of hydrotherapy and electric baking and massage.

ILLUSTRATIVE CASE *Case XXVIII.* (Infectious arthritis.) (From a report by Dr. Proctor.) The patient, a young girl, aged twenty-one, had always been in very good health. As a child she had mumps and measles. Has not had scarlet fever, diphtheria, or pneumonia. Eleven years ago the patient suffered considerably from nasal catarrh, with sore throat and swelling on the side of the neck. This was operated on and discharged for three or four months. Has not been subject to colds or sore throats since; the swelling on the neck did not recur. No tuberculosis or arthritis or carcinoma in the family history.

On Sunday, August 16, 1914, the patient had an ulcerated tooth (right upper central incisor) which was giving her some trouble. The following morning the pain had increased and the face was swollen. She went to the dentist to have it attended to. He lanced an abscess on the gum and gave her another appointment for the following Friday, August 21. During the interval between these visits the girl suffered very great pain and could not sleep nights. The dentist, however, filled the tooth with a gold filling and told the girl that she would have to expect more or less pain, but that the swelling would soon go away. When she went home from this visit her face was so swollen that her mother hardly knew her. After four or five days the face started to become normal and at the same time the left ankle began to get stiff, and shortly afterward the right ankle became affected, then the elbows and thumbs became stiff and swollen. The joints had not been particularly tender, but the condition showed a tendency to steady progression until the patient could hardly walk on account of stiffness and pain. The first physician who took care of her thought that her trouble might be due to a run-down condition, and as she grew gradually worse under his treatment (she saw him two or three times for ten weeks), she was advised to consult another physician, who diagnosed her case as infectious arthritis, with the abscessed tooth as the causative factor. He sent her to the Rhode Island Hospital, where she was admitted November 28, 1914. Physical examination showed nose and throat negative, heart in good condition, lungs clear. Abdomen no masses, no tenderness. On December 22, the jaws started to get stiff, especially the right side, so that her eating was limited to well chopped or soft solid foods. On December 28, the terminal joints of the thumbs were swollen and a dull grating was produced on manipulating the joint. In March, 1915, the patient went home; at this time the girl was perfectly helpless and unable to feed herself; she had to stay in bed. Dr. Painter, who saw the patient in December, 1915, found all the larger joints involved and the small joints of the hands. She was unable to sit up and could not move any of her joints without a great amount of pain. Figure 171 shows a radiograph of her fingers; Figure 172 shows the condition of the devitalized tooth. Dr. Painter ordered massage, regulated the diet; Dr. Proctor performed apiectomy on the upper central incisor on December 24, and removed the scar tissue, which yielded a streptococcus staphylococcus culture. The patient improved very much during the following three months, she was able to get up and go about, the mouth could be opened wider. In April she took cold and had a relapse. Dr. Proctor operated on her again on April 17, having better access to the mouth at this time. The root of the right lateral incisor, which was found devitalized, was amputated, and at the same time he removed the left lower third molar and second bicuspid, which showed abscessed condition. The patient improved again and is now able to sit up in a chair.

Case XXIX. Atrophic arthritis. Patient, a housewife, of sixty-nine years, was admitted to the Robert B. Brigham Hospital on July 3, 1914. Had had measles, pertussis, scarlet fever and lung fever, when a child. Her present illness started two years previous. Both hands became swollen. This swelling was white and painless; later the feet became affected, and the eyes were inflamed. The process subsided slowly and she had not wholly recovered when a second attack was suffered one year before entering the hospital. This time the hands, shoulders, neck and knees were affected and she has not recovered from this attack. Examination showed pupils equal and of normal reaction, tonsils not enlarged, throat negative. No glandular enlargement in neck, axillae or groin. Lungs negative, heart action irregular and systolic murmurs heard at apex and transmitted to axilla. Spleen not palpable, kidneys not palpable, abdomen soft and full, no masses nor tenderness.

Diagnosis: Infectious arthritis with atrophic changes. The patient received house diet and was kept in bed on account of the cardiac condition. X-rays of joints were taken. X-rays of intestine with bismuth meal were taken. The knees, elbows, and hands showed atrophic changes. These were contracted so as to make the patient appear as bent over.

On October 2 the patient was ordered to the hydrotherapy room for electric treatment. On April 29, 1915,

PLATE LV

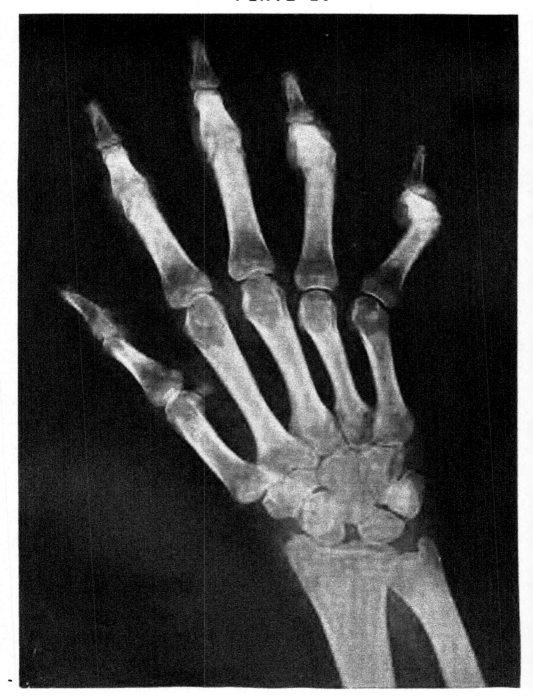

FIG. 171

FIG. 171.—Radiographic plates of one hand of Case No. 28, showing atrophic destruction of several joints. Note the periarticular swelling.

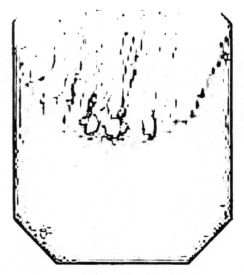

FIG. 172

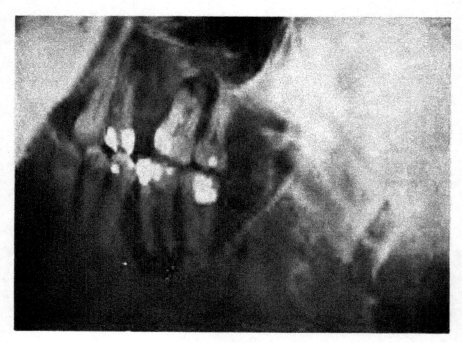

FIG. 173

FIG. 172.—Radiograph showing the bone changes about the incisor which originally had caused the infectious arthritis of Case No. 28, the radiograph had been
taken about sixteen months after the patient had acute symptoms.

FIG. 173.—Radiographic plate of Case No. 29, showing areas of disease about the
roots of the upper first molar and lower first and second molars.

X-rays of her teeth were taken and showed areas of bone absorption on the upper left first molar and the upper right second bicuspid. There were also large areas on the left lower first and second molars, and the right lower second molar. (Figure 173.)

I extracted the teeth and curetted the abscess cavities. After two weeks the patient had more motion in the fingers and wrists, although there were still areas of swelling and tenderness. Soon after, walking for a few steps was successfully attempted. Improvement continued, and after three months she was able to walk up and down stairs, and made considerable gain in the use of her fingers on the piano. At the time of writing, May, 1916, she is in good condition, up every day, eats and sleeps well, walks every day, and has considerable motion in her fingers. She will leave the hospital shortly.

CHAPTER IX

EXAMINATION OF THE ORAL CAVITY

The mode of examination of the mouth is perhaps today the greatest shortcoming of the average dentist. The patient who trusts his family dentist entirely takes it for granted that the dentist's examination is complete and thorough, and believes that the mouth has been restored to a normal and healthy condition when being dismissed. The radiologist's examination reveals many unsuspected abscesses in the mouths of patients, to whose mouths dentists have given conscientious if mistaken attention. It often takes a good deal of explanation to righten the dentist's position in such cases and to sooth the patient's anger at having been deceived. While the dentist, of course, is not to blame for conditions which have been caused and have developed without his knowledge, the situation must be properly explained. The patient will be quick to realize that the dentist had only the best intentions in trying to save every tooth as an important organ of mastication and that he surely is not to blame for not having been able to accomplish the impossible in correctly treating many abnormally developed teeth and obstructed root canals, and for not knowing that such dangerous septic conditions can exist in his patient's mouth without giving any symptoms. But today, with our modern means of examination, where X-ray machines are especially adapted for our purposes and where radiologists are to be found in almost every street, where there are professional men, there is no excuse for a dentist to neglect to ascertain the condition of all devitalized teeth in his patient's mouth. But he who only fills cavities, constructs bridges and makes

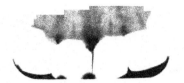

FIG. 174

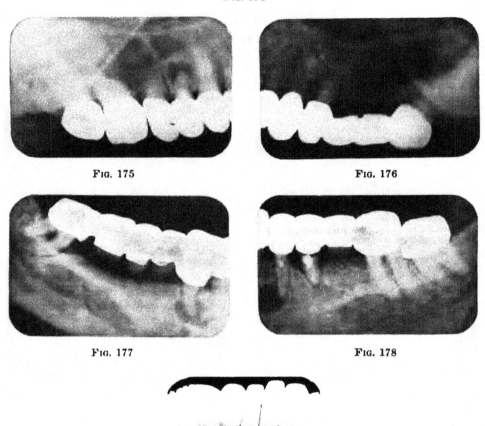

FIG. 175

FIG. 176

FIG. 177

FIG. 178

FIG. 179

FIG. 174, 175, 176, 177, 178 and 179.—Radiographs of a mouth showing a large amount of crown and bridge work of recent date and a great many abscess areas.

PLATE LVIII

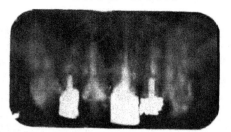

FIG. 180

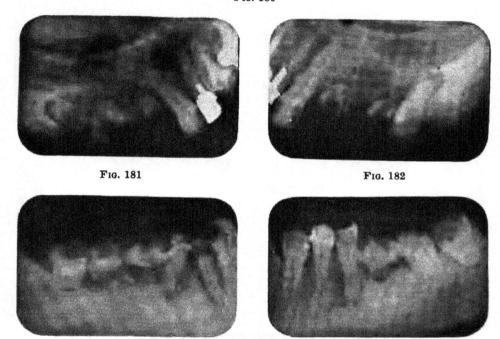

FIG. 181   FIG. 182

FIG. 183   FIG. 184

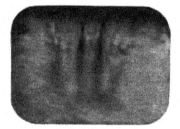

FIG. 185

FIGS. 180, 181, 182, 183, 184 and 185.—Radiographs of a neglected mouth showing broken-down teeth and abscess areas.

plates and neglects other abnormal or diseased conditions which the patient does not particularly complain of, renders poor service to the public. The dentist is the man who has charge of the mouth and he has a great responsibility. It would put the dental profession back to the age of the mechanic should we undertake to concern ourselves only with mechanical restoration instead of investigating and treating every disease found in the region of our domain. What would we think of an ophthalmologist who would only correct abnormal conditions of the lens and would pay no attention to co-existing iritis or other inflammatory diseases of the eye? But we find exactly parallel cases in the practice of many dentists.

METHOD OF ORAL EXAMINATION FOR THE PHYSICIAN The physician often has occasion to inquire into the condition of his patient's mouth, especially when in search of a focus or foci of the disease concerning which the patient is consulting him. Some medical men still have the idea that the mouth is a thing apart from the body which cannot have any influence upon the general health, others are too easily satisfied with the patient's statement that the dentist is visited regularly and that there is absolutely nothing wrong with the teeth, but the thorough physician will not be satisfied except with a report based upon a careful examination and radiographic diagnosis made by a dentist or radiologist in whose judgment he can trust.

A superficial examination of the mouth by the physician should include the following:

1. *Examination of the soft tissues of the mouth.* The tongue, floor of the mouth, palate and gums should be inspected. Stomatitis is easily detectable and in pyorrhoea the gums are inflamed and spongy, and pus can be squeezed out from underneath the gum.

2. *Examination of the teeth. Neglected teeth* can be recognized at a glance; there are many cavities and broken down teeth causing abscesses with or without visible sinuses on the gum.

Overdentristried teeth are of a most deceiving nature. Teeth of dark appearance, gold and porcelain crowns and bridges always come under suspicion, because these are generally signs of devitalized teeth, and it makes no difference whether the gums are inflamed or normal, with no sinus, and no symptoms of inflammation whatever. Radiographs should be secured of such teeth as this is the only means of finding out their condition.

Impacted and unerupted teeth should be investigated by the X-ray. If some teeth are missing and the patient does not remember that they were extracted it is possible that they are in malposition and cause disturbance.

3. *Enlarged Lymph Glands.* If the submental or sub-maxillary lymph glands are enlarged, it is almost always a sign that some septic process is going on in the mouth. Abscesses, however, may occur without the involvement of the glands.

METHOD OF ORAL EXAMINATION FOR THE DENTIST The old method of dental examination has already been criticized in the first part of this chapter. But worse than the method of examination is the way the dentist keeps his records. The card systems and books which are on the market are absolutely inefficient, for besides a place for bookkeeping they provide only for records of the fillings placed in the teeth and the crowns and bridges made for the patient. There is no arrangement that provides for the marking of root canal operations, for indicating abscess and pyorrhoea conditions, not to speak of other diseases which may be directly or indirectly connected with the conditions found in the oral cavity.

The dentist should inquire into, examine and record the following conditions:

PHYSICAL EXAMINATION 1. *General Health of the Patient.* The dentist should inquire into the general condition of the patient's health and if a history of systemic disease is found in connection with septic processes of the mouth, the patient should be en-

PLATE LIX

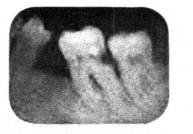

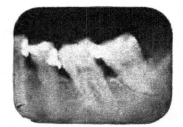

FIG. 186

FIG. 187

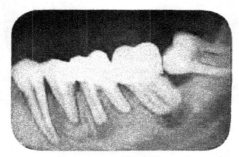

FIG. 188

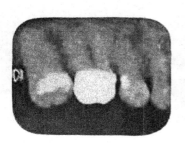

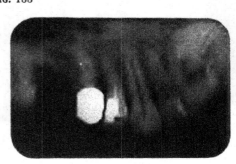

FIG. 189

FIG. 190

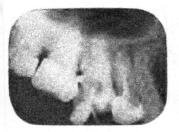

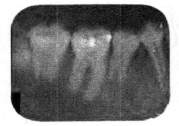

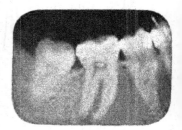

FIG. 191

FIG. 192

FIG. 193

FIGS. 186 and 187.—Radiographs revealing deep cavities causing obscure pain. Both on the distal side of the first molar.

FIG. 188.—Radiograph shows a large amount of unsuspected trouble.

FIGS. 189, 190, 191, 192 and 193.—Radiographs showing the value of X-rays before undertaking root canal work. In Fig. 189 note bent apex of second bicuspid with gold crown. In Fig. 191, cuspid with root bent at right angle. In Fig. 192, the foramina of some teeth are still widely open. In Fig. 193 there is a pulp stone in the pulp chamber of the first molar.

PLATE LX

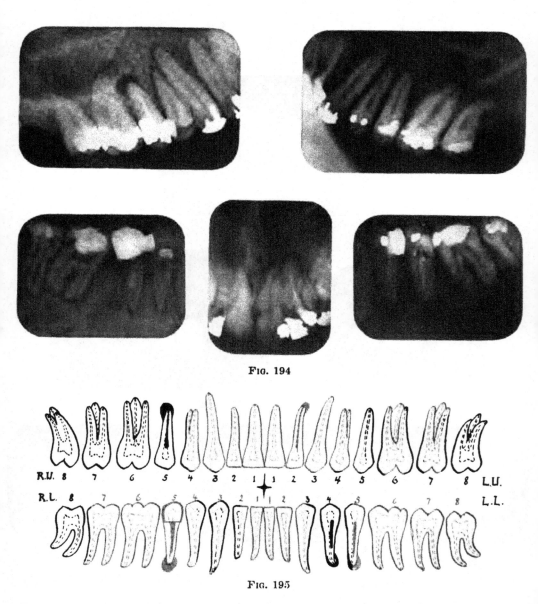

FIG. 194

FIG. 195

FIGS. 194 and 195.—Radiographs of a mouth which was examined for foci and report chart indicating the granulomata and root canal fillings.

couraged to consult a physician, whose coöperation should be secured to find out whether there is any connection between the two conditions and what further treatment besides the treatment of the oral condition could be of benefit to the patient.

2. *Diseases of the Soft Tissues.* The tongue, palate, floor of the mouth and gums should be examined next. Abscesses, ulcers, cancers, gummata, palatal perforations and clefts, benign and malignant tumors, cysts, diseases of the salivary glands and ducts, inflammation of the throat, stomatitis and pyorrhœa may be noticed.

3. *Diseases of the Teeth.* Malocclusion should be noticed in children, missing teeth and lack of masticating efficiency in adults. Cavities may be in plain view or may only be discovered after most careful exploration. If the patient complains of pain the teeth should be tested to find out diseased conditions of the pulp. Applications of ice or hot instruments to the various teeth, as well as the galvanic or high frequency current are useful aids to diagnosis. Acute periodontitis is recognized if a tooth is tender and pain is caused on percussion, acute abscesses and parulis are noticed in like manner, the latter causing noticeable swelling of the face and gum. Sinuses on the gum without complaint of pain and tenderness lead to chronic abscesses caused by devitalized teeth, and all devitalized teeth whether they cause apparent trouble or not should be recognized; these are usually darker in appearance, have large fillings or large cavities, porcelain crowns or gold crowns which may also serve as abutment of bridges. Such teeth should be radiographed to find out the periapical condition and the quality of the root canal fillings. Finally, the dentist should be on the lookout for impacted and unerupted teeth, which usually sooner or later become a source of serious trouble. In children they may cause malocclusion; in adults, various abnormal and diseased conditions, as we have already seen.

RADIO-GRAPHIC EXAMINATION It is impossible to make a thorough examination of the mouth without the use of radiographs in patients who have devitalized teeth. If the dentist has not an X-ray machine of his own, he can easily secure radiographs of the suspected teeth from a dental radiologist, who will not only take the radiographs, but will also give valuable advice as to the interpretation of the pictures. It is indeed a great advantage to be able to consult a man who as a specialist sees many cases and therefore has a much greater experience in radiographic diagnosis than the general practitioner, and the fee for such services with the modern improvements has been reduced to a level which is in the realm of almost every person.

Radiographs are principally taken to find obscure causes, to ascertain physical diagnosis, to diagnose obscure conditions, to prognose the outcome of therapeutic measures, the possibilities of treatment and the course of surgical technique.

1. *Obscure pain* may be diagnosed by means of radiographs and found to come from decay under the gingival margin or under fillings, from impacted and unerupted teeth or cysts and acute abscesses.

2. *Diagnosis of Condition of Devitalized Teeth.* The use of radiographs to find out the conditions of pulpless teeth has revolutionized the attitude towards devitalization of teeth. It made us realize the difficulty and value of good root canal fillings and the consequences of neglect and inability to perform perfect root canal work. Radiographs show whether the root fillings reach the apex or whether the canal is only filled part way. Broken root-canal instruments are detected as well as perforations at the side. The apex may show a ragged appearance, which is a sign of necrosis of the root; or it may appear enlarged and bulging on account of exostosis of the cementum. There may be an area of lessened density around the apex showing loss of bone; this indicates an abscessed condition or a granuloma. Similar areas occur sometimes on the

PLATE LXI

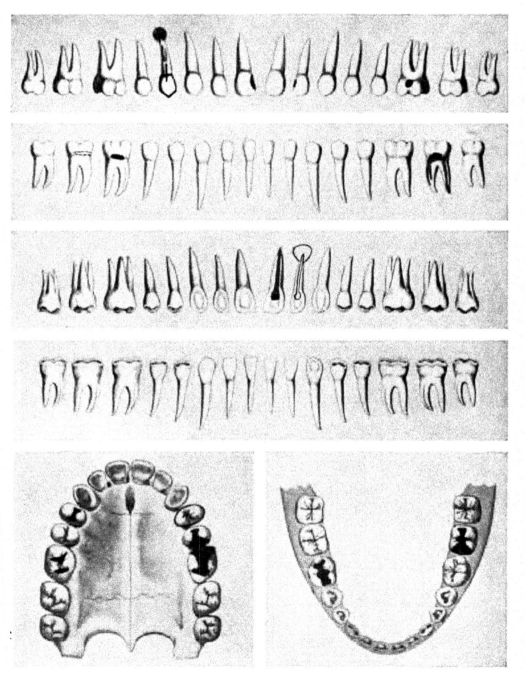

FIG. 196.—Record chart as used by Dr. Potter and reproduced with his permission.

side of a root or between the roots of multirooted teeth. There may also be absorption of bone at the cervical part of the alveolar process surrounding the bone, indicating pus pocket.

3. *Prognosis Before Root Canal Treatment.* It is of great importance to make sure of the probable outcome before involving the patient in lengthy and expensive root canal treatment. The radiograph may show normal canals, open apical foramina, accessory foramina, bent and curved roots, inacessible canals on account of secondary dentine, pulp stones or broken root-canal instruments. Abscess formation and necrosis of the apex may be discovered which would indicate the necessity of surgical interference and generally gives an idea whether a tooth can be saved or not, whether the root canals can be treated with medicines, and the canal filled to the apex, whether apiectomy is practical and indicated to save the tooth or whether the tooth has to be extracted.

POTTER CASE CHARTS
All these findings should be recorded on a chart. Professor William H. Potter, who realized the shortcomings of the ordinary dentist's examination charts, took much pains in arranging a practical chart on which all dental conditions can be marked down. Figure 196 shows an examination recorded on his chart. The plates also have historic interest: they are copies of originals from Carabelli*. The back of the chart is arranged for book-keeping.

Similar but simpler charts have been made up by the author for reports of radiographic examination. This is sent with the radiographs and gives the dentist a better idea and clearer picture of the condition of the whole mouth, which can be verified by the radiographs. In this chart the radiologist can interpret the radiographic findings so that they are plainly visible. Such a chart is seen in Figure 195.

---

* CARABELLI: Die Anatomie des Mundes.

CHAPTER X

TREATMENT OF ORAL ABSCESSES

The treatment of oral abscesses varies with the anatomical location and with the condition of the inflammation. The treatments of the various conditions will be discussed under the following headings:

1. Treatment of acute and subacute conditions.
2. Treatment of chronic conditions.
3. Treatment of abscesses due to diseases of the gums.
4. Treatment of abscesses from impacted and unerupted teeth.
5. Treatment of abscesses of the tongue.
6. Treatment of abscesses of the salivary glands and ducts.
7. Treatment of systemic conditions.

1. *Treatment of Acute and Subacute Conditions.*

In treating acute conditions we should carefully differentiate between acute and subacute inflammation. In acute inflammation, especially in the beginning stage where there is little destruction of tissue, the tissue reacts easily to treatment and complete regeneration is possible. In subacute cases, however, a chronic condition has previously existed, the root may be necrosed, and the reaction of the tissue is therefore not sufficient to produce complete recovery when the acute symptoms subside. The inflammation passes back into the quiescent and persistent chronic stage. It is therefore important to diagnose the cause correctly, and distinguish between the acute condition which occurred as a primary infection of the periapical tissue, from an infected pulp, and the subacute condition, which can be recognized by the history or by a radiograph showing that the root canal had been treated or filled previously. In the subacute cases, extraction is indicated unless the conditions are favorable for apiectomy, but before this operation can be performed, the same treatment is indicated as for the acute conditions until the symptoms quiet down, when the tooth can be filled and surgically treated.

REMOVAL OF THE CAUSE Acute periodontitis sometimes can be stopped and extensive alveolar abscess prevented by prompt removal of the cause. In the later stages of acute abscess it is of equal importance to eliminate the causative factor, which is a suppurating pulp. When opening into the tooth use a good sized round burr, holding the tooth firmly by making a plaster cast for each side, so as to decrease the jarring and to prevent further irritation. If there is much pain, conductive or general anaesthesia is indicated. Remove the largest part of the pulp in a gentle manner so as not to press infected material through the apical foramen. If the radiograph indicates that abscess formation has already begun, it may be advisable to enlarge the root canal and apical foramen so as to get reasonably free access to the abscess. All this is done under aseptic precautions. A mild antiseptic dressing is placed into the tooth, such as:

Buckley's Modified phenol:
    Mentholis ....gr. xx
    Thymolis ....gr. xl
    Phenolis ....F3 iij MX

Black recommends:
    Ol. cassiae ....1 part
    Phenolis ....2 parts
    Ol. gaultheriae ....3 parts
Mx oils and add melted crystals of phenol.

Close the opening of the tooth with cotton dipped in liquid petroleum; this prevents saliva from entering, but allows gases which may be formed in the canals to escape. Change the dressing daily until the tooth feels more comfortable, when the dressing can be sealed into the tooth with base plate gutta percha. After the root canals have been cleaned and sterilized, they should be filled, so as to seal the apical foramina hermetically. Only by scrupulous asepsis, careful treatment and technique can recurrence or chronic continuation be prevented. This technique will be described in the chapter on prevention.

REST OF THE DISE SED TOOTH To avoid further irritation the affected elongated tooth should be put at rest. This is best done by building up the occlusial surface of all the teeth of one jaw with copper cement except in the position of the tender tooth.

APPLICATION OF COUNTER-IRRITANTS Counter-irritants are beneficial to help absorb the abscess. Apply on both sides of the gum, over the affected root, tincture of iodine, tincture of iodine and aconite, or chloroform; these are the most common counter-irritants. They should be applied to the dried mucous membrane. Suction cups containing counter-irritants are applied on the gum opposite the apex of the root.

ALVEO-LATOMY In some cases of acute abscess, we can gain sufficient drainage through the root canal to affect a cure. This is true for upper teeth if treatment is started before the destructive process has progressed too far. In lower teeth this is almost impossible, because the process is not aided by gravitation. The abscess in the mandible is also of much more severe nature, more pain is produced, and a longer time is required, because of anatomical conditions, till the pus burrows an opening through the bone to the surface. Great relief and good drainage can be secured by an artificial opening through the alveolar process. Under conductive or general anaesthesia we incise the gum, retract it to both sides, and with a large round burr drill through the process to the apex of the tooth. The opening should be made at the lowest level. The root canal can be opened at a future sitting, though I prefer to do it at once. If the apical foramen can be penetrated, irrigation through the tooth is indicated. Normal salt or mild antiseptic solution should be used. Put a mild antiseptic dressing into the tooth, as already described, and a wick into the artificial sinus to prevent premature closing of the wound. I prefer to use a cigarette wick made of rubber tissue; this does not disintegrate. The abscess should be irrigated daily until no more pus is discharged, when the root canal can be filled. The wound should heal from the bottom; this is accomplished by shortening the wick. If suppuration persists we must ascertain the cause. Usually this comes from necrosis of the tooth and can only be cured by amputation of the diseased part.

In cases presenting a subperiosteal or subgingival parulis, an early incision will quickly relieve the pain. The pus, which has already penetrated the outer plate of the bone and collected in large quantity under the periosteum or gum, cannot be expected to drain back through the bone and root canal of the tooth. Therefore we should at once, under conductive or general anaesthesia, secure a large incision at as low a level as possible. In case of subperiosteal parulis, which is particularly liable to cause extensive necrosis, especially if it is of long duration, this incision should be very extensive so as to give free drainage. Some authors recommend leaving the tooth alone until the acute symptoms have subsided, but I prefer to remove the cause at once. If conductive or general anaesthesia is used, this may be effected when the abscess is incised. An opening should be drilled into the tooth and the bulk of the diseased pulp is removed. The incision is made on the gum as described. The pus should be taken up with a sponge, especially under general anaesthesia. The point of a piston syringe or fountain syringe is inserted into the root canal and the whole area is washed out thoroughly with normal salt or mild antiseptic solution. Under general anaesthesia this solution should be taken up by sponges and not left to run into the mouth.

Under conductive anaesthesia the management is much simpler and the whole treatment can be done more successfully. The incision should be kept open by means of a wick made of rubber tissue, and the washing should be repeated until the discharge of pus stops. The opening in the tooth can be closed temporarily after an antiseptic dressing has been placed into the root canal. After the root canal has been cleaned and sterilized it can be filled, and if this is correctly done, the abscess will not recur or continue as a chronic lesion unless the periodontal membrane has been destroyed at the apex of the root or become necrosed during the period of suppuration. In such cases we have to resort to apiectomy or extraction.

EXTRACTION The most radical, but usually also the quickest relief is extraction of the offending tooth. If the patient's resistance is low so that a speedy healing by the application of any one of the above methods cannot be expected, or, if high fever or complications set in, it is almost always advisable to resort to more radical means. If extraction is decided upon, it should be undertaken at once, because nothing is gained by waiting. It is an erroneous idea that a tooth should not be extracted during the acute stage. Nothing gives a more spontaneous result than elimination of the cause and establishment of drainage through the alveolar socket. The extraction should be performed under general or local conductive anaesthesia. Spray the mouth thoroughly and paint the tooth and surrounding gum with iodine to prevent secondary infection. The extraction should be followed by curettage, after which the wound is freely irrigated, treated with iodine, and lightly packed with gauze. Antiseptics and anodines can be applied on this dressing; iodoform, orthoform, or the following preparation is of benefit:

Euroform paste:
    Orthoform 40
    Europhen 60
Add liquid petroleum to make a paste.

The wound should be irrigated daily and granulation should be allowed to fill the cavity from the bottom. An antiseptic mouth wash should be used freely and often and held in the mouth for five to ten minutes at a time. If the socket does not fill in with granulation tissue speedily it is advisable to procure a slight hemorrhage with a sterilized instrument. The socket is then filled with a blood clot which organizes in a very short time. In cases where the disease has progressed to the stage of parulis, an incision should be made on the gum in addition to the extraction and communication established from the gum to the socket. Curette the diseased process and irrigate profusely. The socket is treated with tincture of iodine placed into the wound of the gum to drain the abscess and permit the socket to fill in with a blood clot. The dressing is changed every day until suppuration is stopped, when the wound is left to heal.

SYSTEMIC TREATMENT *For Palliative Effect.* A hot foot-bath and cathartic should be ordered. Prescribe the foot-bath as follows: A tub is partly filled with warm water and the feet immersed. Hotter water is added to raise the temperature of the bath to the greatest degree that can be tolerated. Powdered mustard may be dissolved in warm water and added to the foot-bath. (Do not dissolve the powder directly in the hot water; it would defeat the action necessary to produce the irritant volatile oil.) Keep the feet in the water five to ten minutes. The effect is dilation of the blood vessels in the lower extremities, reducing the blood pressure in the head. After the foot-bath the feet should be thoroughly dried and the patient should go to bed, which has been warmed beforehand. It is essential not to step on a cold floor with the bare feet, or to chill the feet in any way, because this would contract the vessels again and spoil the effect.

For a cathartic prescribe castor oil in gelatine capsules. Six $2\frac{1}{2}$ gram capsules should be taken before retiring.

Other laxatives are:

Tab. Cascara Sagrada a.a. 0.3 chocolate coated.
Sig.   One to two tablets before retiring.

or,

Aloini ... ...gr. 1/5
Strychnia   ....gr. 1/120
Ext. Belladonna Fol...........gr. 0/8

S.   Take one to two pills before retiring.

An alternative may also be given in certain cases:

℞

Potassii iodidi ....6.0 g. — 3 jss.
Syrupi sarsaparillae comp. 90.0—f3 iij.

Sig.   Take a teaspoonful in water every 2 hours
till 3 doses are taken, then a teaspoonful after meals.

For Relief of Pain.   Phenacetin and aspirin have
been found by the author the most effective antipyretic
for pain in the trigeminal region.   Give gr. V of each and
repeat after one hour if necessary.   Trigeminin gr. V or
pyramidon gr. II s.s. sometimes prove of value.   To tide
the patient over a very severe attack or to give a night's
rest a hypnotic may be used.   Tab. Bromural (Knoll &
Co.) a.a. 0.3 (gr. V) two to three tablets before retiring
should be given.   In extreme cases:

℞

Morphiae sulph........0.015   gr. ¼
Kalii Bromid. ....2.0   gr. xxx
Aquae ....30.0   3 i

Sig.   One half to be taken at once; balance in three
hours, if needed.

For prompt relief give ⅛ or ¼ gr. morphine hypodermically.

Diet.   Order a light, easily digestible diet which is
strengthening at the same time.

TREATMENT OF SINUS TO FACE If a sinus to the face exists we always have to resort to extraction of the responsible tooth. The discharging of an abscess in the face is often invited by poultices or hot applications to the face. This should be avoided; poultices if used should be applied to the gum and cold applications only to the face. If a sinus exists it should be curetted and washed. After extraction of the tooth and curetting of the diseased area the sinus will close up speedily; unfortunately, however, not without leaving a permanent mark. This scar can be improved somewhat by excision of the fibrous connection which fixes the skin to the bone and closing of the wound by a plastic operation.

2. *Treatment of Chronic Condition.*

Chronic abscesses in all stages are of very persistent character and the fact that they cause none of the cardinal symptoms makes it extremely hard to ascertain in a general way whether the lesion is yielding to treatment or not. Even the radiograph for this special purpose is not always a safe means of finding out, because lighter and darker shadows, smaller and larger areas can be obtained by variation in the exposure, the quality of the ray, the depth of the development and the angle at which the exposure is made. Generally we may say that as long as there is any area of lessened density at all and as long as the root end is necrosed we cannot claim to have cured the abscess.

Antiseptic treatment of chronic abscesses has for a long time been the treatment *per se.* A large number of drugs have been and still are in use. They are either forced through the apical foramen but more frequently are only applied into the root canal of the tooth by means of cotton dressings, and it is left to their power of evaporation to penetrate into the diseased periapical tissue and cure the abscess. Ionic medication has been recommended to carry the antiseptic into the diseased tissue. Careful experiments with these methods and a variety of drugs proved to my satisfaction that there is today no antiseptic known that has sufficient penetrating and sterilizing power to destroy bacterial life completely in the periapical granulomata. I have treated blind abscesses of medium size from the root canal with all known methods and found such treatment extremely uncertain, if not entirely insufficient. Grieves,* whom I consider one of the most thorough investigators, makes the following statement about treatment of pericemental conditions: "There is to my knowledge no medicament nor method, germicidal, oxydizing or electrolytic, that will revivify the pericemental apex. If it be vital, the tooth is healthy; if it be diseased, the tooth is next to doomed. This is the point in treatment where materia medica stops and good surgery begins."

This is exactly my opinion, based upon histopathological study, as shown in Chapter VI, and investigations especially undertaken to study the value of the different popular methods of medication.

Original Investigation of the Efficiency of Medication for the Treatment of Granulomata.

Five teeth in different patients have been used for experiments. All cases showed an area of about pea size and were of long standing. I first used antiseptic dressings until there was no more odor. Teeth 1 and 2 received no further treatment. Teeth 3 and 4 received zinc ions, milliampere for ten minutes on two different days, the fifth tooth received iodine ions ½ to 1 milliampere for fifteen minutes on two days. Tooth 1 was extracted; on tooth 2 apiectomy was performed. Cultures were made both from root apex and abscess and showed bacterial growth. Tooth 3 was extracted. No growth from the root apex, slight bacterial growth from the abscess. Apiectomy was undertaken on tooth 4 and bac-

* GRIEVES, C. J.: Dental Periapical Infection as the Cause of Systemic Disease. *Dental Cosmos*, January, 1914.

terial growth was received from both abscess and root. Tooth 5 was also a case of root amputation; the abscess yielded a culture of staphylococcus albus and a few very small chains of streptococci.

Another case showed the inefficiency of ionic medication in the treatment of the chronic abscess; Mr. R. suffered with arthritis and especially complained of toxemia and decreased mental capacity. He had to stop smoking as the system was not able to take care of the nicotine. From radiographic examination I concluded that there were chronic abscesses on left upper first and second bicuspids and proliferating periodontitis on the left upper cuspid. The root canals were carefully cleaned and treated with medicines, zinc ions were used twice and iodine ions once, then I filled the canals. Much care was taken in condensing the root canal fillings which resulted in forcing the root canal cones through the foramina. During the treatment the patient received great relief and finally got rid of the systemic conditions, his head was clear in the morning, and he was especially pleased that he could again smoke "like a chimney." After five or six months he returned, however, saying that his old symptoms were returning. I delayed treatment for four or five weeks longer, when he was almost as bad as before. Radiographs showed about the same amount of decreased density about the two bicuspid roots. Apiectomy was performed and cultures procured. These yielded a bacterial growth and the symptoms disappeared almost entirely several days after the operation.

From these observations I conclude that in cases where we do not deal with a purely local condition, but where the patient's health is involved, more radical treatment than medication is recommendable.

A chronic alveolar abscess or granuloma looked at from the viewpoint of the bone instead of the tooth is, as already mentioned, an osteomyelitic condition; the disease occurs in the bone and at the expense of the bone, and the only reason why the disease does not spread more easily is due to the abundant blood supply of the jaws and the protecting reaction of the tissues which form a fibrous layer at the periphery of the lesion enclosing the seat of suppuration. In cases where there is necrosis of the root, and necrosis occurs in most all roots surrounded for a long time by chronic inflammation, it is impossible to cure the condition without getting rid of the diseased part by surgical means. In cases where the disease has not progressed beyond the apical part, the usual condition, we can separate the necrosed part of the tooth surgically and curette the bone, which will induce prompt healing of the condition. This operation permits us to extirpate the abscess radically, remove the necrosed root end surgically, and still save the tooth.

REMOVAL OF THE CAUSE Also in chronic disease it is imperative to remove the primary cause. The principal cause of proliferating periodontitis and granulomata is the condition of septic and imperfectly filled root canals. Our aim therefore ought to be to thoroughly cleanse the root canal and remove all infected tissue. Root canal treatment and root canal filling are operations which require considerable skill and patience. The technique will be described in the chapter on prevention.

TREATMENT WITH ANTI-SEPTICS PLACED INTO THE ROOT CANAL Antiseptics applied into the root canal have, as already discussed, been used for a long time to render the tooth aseptic. I do not think that they ever were meant to be used for treatment of chronic abscesses, and their insufficiency for this purpose has already been enlarged upon, but it may be wise to say also that formaldehyde, either alone or combined with other drugs, has never been meant to be the cure of all pulp and periapical diseases. Dr. G. V. Black has described at length its irritating action and its power of destroying periodontal membrane, and Buckley himself has stated that formaldehyde acts only on the surface and has no penetrating power.

IONIC MEDICATION Ionic medication is advisable in all those cases of short standing where the proliferation of the periodontal membrane is of small extent and where the apex has not been affected by necrosis nor the periodontal membrane destroyed. The effect of ionic medication is to distribute into the surrounding tissues the antiseptic placed in the root canal. The dentinal tubules, as well as accessory foramina, are sterilized by this method, which prevents later reinfection. The therapeutic action depends on the drug used; zinc, copper, silver, and iodine are most commonly employed.

Zinc Ion. A zinc electrode is used with a three per cent. solution of zinc chloride applied on a few fibres of cotton. Place the zinc broach into the root canal. The positive pole is used in the tooth, the negative pole is held in the hand, or applied to the cheek, and one-half to three milliamperes are applied for from five to fifteen minutes. The action of zinc chloride is tissue destructive. It is used by some men to destroy the granuloma, which is then thought to be resorbed.

Copper Ion. A two per cent. solution of copper sulphate is used with a copper anode on the positive pole. One milliampere seems to give a good dissociation of ions. Its action is similar to zinc chlorid.

Iodine Ion. Tincture of iodine is used and applied on the negative pole, preferably on an iridium platinum electrode. Use one half to three milliamperes for five to fifteen minutes. To be safe the treatment should be repeated.

Action of Antiseptic Ions. The effect of ionic medication is to distribute the antiseptic deeper into the tissues. Its action is destructive to bacteria. The zinc ion seems to be the most effective, but like the copper ion, it seems to have a decidedly irritating and tissue destructive, if not escharotic or caustic effect. Symptoms of swelling and pain have been observed after the treatment in several cases by the author, and for this reason the iodine ions are more commendable. It has only a bactericidal action and does not destroy the tissue, and is well known as the great antiseptic. I have used an aqueous solution of iodine lately. It has all the iodine properties minus the irritating action, and also penetrates more profusely in moist tissue. Ionic medication with iodine is of great importance for root canal sterilization and is to be highly recommended for routine practice to sterilize in a proper way the dentinal tubules and accessory foramina of a tooth, as will be described in the chapter on prevention.

APIECTOMY Apiectomy is an operation by which we can positively eliminate a chronic abscess without sacrificing the tooth. It is the only sure method of treatment if the apex of the root is diseased, if the apical periodontal membrane is destroyed, if the root canal cannot be treated and filled to the very end, if the side of the root has been perforated near the apex by a root-canal instrument, or if an instrument has been broken off in the end of the root. It can also be performed on teeth that carry crowns or bridges if the root canal is accessible and properly treated and filled previous to the operation. Not all teeth, however, are favorable cases. The operation is impossible on third and almost always on second molars. The first molars are frequently accessible, and all the remaining teeth can easily be operated upon.

The operation consists in opening through the side of the alveolar process, amputation and removal of the diseased root apex and thorough curettage of the diseased bone. It is a strictly aseptic surgical operation.

Radiographic examination: A careful examination of the condition of the occlusion and a study of the length and shape of the root by means of a good radiograph is imperative. The condition of the root canal should be investigated; from the radiograph we can judge how well we shall be able to fill it. Observe also the position of the neighboring teeth and how much alveolar process to hold the tooth there will be left after the operation. A tooth with pyorrhoea or with an apical periodontitis extending almost to the alveolar border is not a favorable case, be-

PLATE LXII

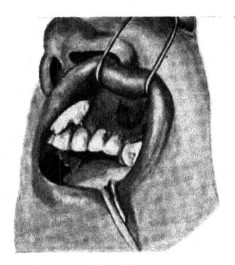

FIG. 197

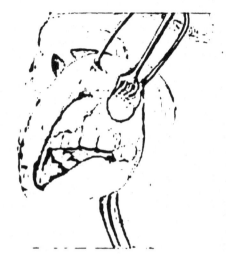

FIG. 198

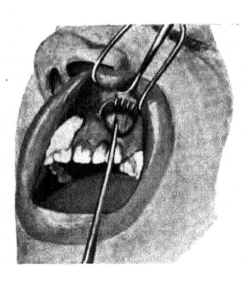

FIG. 199

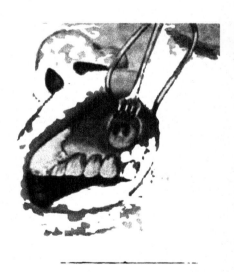

FIG. 200

FIGS. 197, 198, 199 and 200.— Apiectomy, on the left upper cuspid. Fig. 197 shows incision,
Fig. 198 gum and periosteum retracted, Fig. 199, cutting of a window into the alveolar process
to expose the root end, Fig. 200, the root end and granuloma exposed.

PLATE LXIII

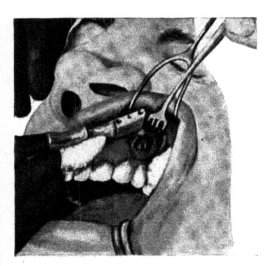

FIG. 201

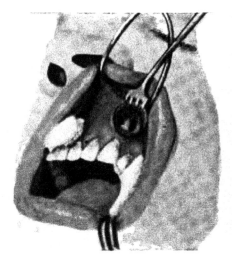

FIG. 202

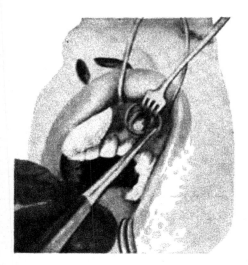

FIG. 203

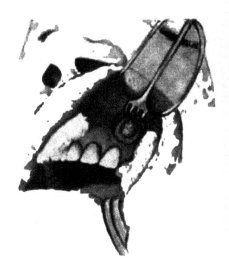

FIG. 204

FIGS. 201, 202, 203 and 204.—Apicetomy continued. Fig. 201 shows the amputation of the diseased root apex with fissure burr. Fig. 202 shows the root end separated. Fig. 203 shows its removal, and Fig. 204 shows the clean bone cavity after the diseased bone has been curetted.

PLATE LXIV

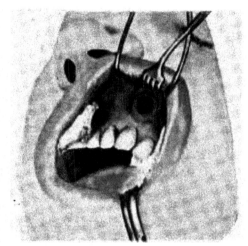

FIG. 205

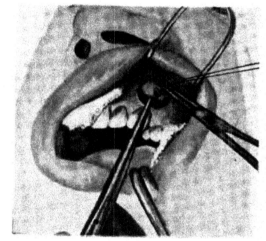

FIG. 206

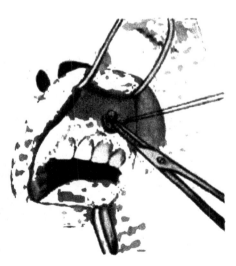

FIG. 207

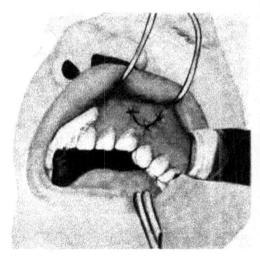

FIG. 208

FIGS. 205, 206, 207 and 208.—Apiectomy continued. Fig. 205, bleeding has been stimulated so as to fill in the bone cavity. Figs. 206 and 207 show the first horse-hair suture. Fig. 208 shows the completed operation.

cause after the operation there would not be enough
periodontal membrane or bone left to give firm attachment to the tooth; neither should a tooth be operated on
if the tooth next to it has also a chronic abscess which
will either directly or indirectly reinfect the healing
tissue.

Treatment of the Root Canal. Apiectomy is only successful if the root canal has been sterilized and properly
filled previous to the operation. It is not sufficient
simply to amputate the root where the old filling ends; but
the root canal and dentinal tubules have to be sterilized,
or there will be reinfection from the tubules exposed
where the root is cut. If it is not worth while to remove
a crown and treat the root canal, the tooth should be extracted or there will be recurrence (with or without
symptoms) and the patient is as badly off as before. It
is not justifiable to leave a crown on a tooth because it is
a masterpiece of art, if the foundation upon which it is
built ruins the patient's health. The root canal should
be rendered aseptic by application of antiseptics or by
ionic medication. It should be filled with the rosin-chlo-
roform-gutta-percha method, which has the advantage
of making the point adhere firmly to the root canal. Dr.
William H. Potter, Professor of Operative Dentistry,
Harvard University Dental School, inserts root canal
fillings with pure lead points. That pure lead is accep-
table to the tissue has been proven by the encapsulation
of bullets in almost any part of the body. It has the
advantage of being burnishable from the abscess cavity,
of not disintegrating, and of safely staying in place during root-canal reaming for fitting of a post and crown. I
use the following method for lead fillings: Dehydrate the
root canal with acetone and hot air, dry with electric root
canal dryer until the patient feels the heat. Fill chloroform and resin (dram I to gr. IV) with a sub-Q syringe
into the canal and insert a gutta-percha point or cone,
pumping it forty times up and down. Remove the remains of the point and insert a lead cone, previously sterilized by boiling it or immersing it for five minutes into

phenol and five minutes into alcohol. Condense the filling as well as possible with root filling condensers so that it adapts itself to the walls. Any filling or crowning of the tooth is performed before the operation so as not to disturb the healing process.

Preparing the Patient for the Operation. If local anaesthesia is used, it sometimes is necessary to use preoperative treatment, especially in nervous, apprehensive, and hysteric patients. Bromural-Knoll (alphabromisovaleryl urea) is an excellent sedative; one tablet is given to children, two to adults (in water thirty minutes before the operation), or $\frac{1}{4}$ gram of morphia hypodermically one hour before the operation.

Preparing the Field of Operation. The mouth should be sprayed out with an antiseptic solution, and the mucous membrane should be cleaned with a cotton roll in the area where we intend to operate.

Anaesthesia. Local anaesthesia, applied by the improved technique* with novocain suprarenin is best adapted for this operation. The amount of suprarenin should not be too large, because too much local anaemia is undesirable, making it almost impossible to procure enough hemorrhage at the end of the operation to fill the bone cavity with blood.

Radiograph. A new intraoral radiograph can be taken at this stage, while we wait for the anaesthesia to take effect. This is essential to ascertain the extent of the root canal filling.

Preparation for the Operation. The operation should be performed on the principles of aseptic surgery. The instruments have been selected beforehand, have been boiled and put on a sterile table, and are covered with a sterile towel until they are used. A sterile table is prepared to deposit the instruments for use, the patient is covered with a sterile sheet, and in order to exclude the hair, the head is covered with a sterile towel except over

---

* *See* THOMA: Textbook on Oral Anaesthesia.

PLATE LXV

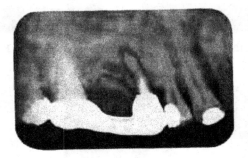

FIG. 209

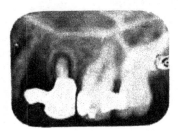

FIG. 210

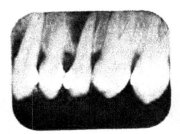

FIG. 211

FIGS. 209, 210 and 211.—Radiographs of three cases which are not favorable for apiectomy because the bone and periodontal membrane has been diseased from the apex to the neck of the tooth.

PLATE LXVI

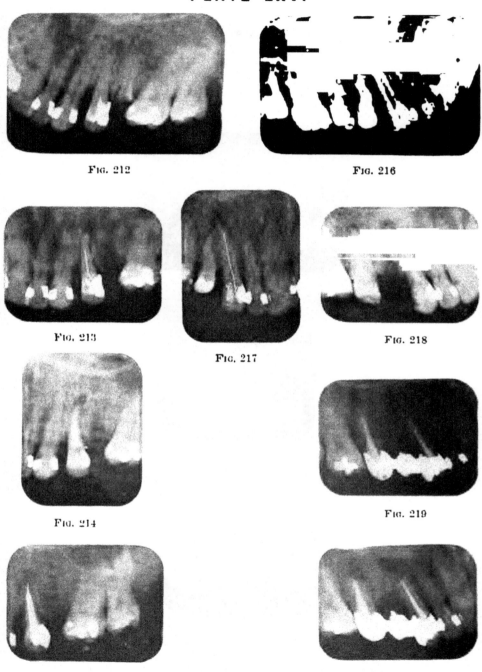

FIG. 212

FIG. 216

FIG. 213

FIG. 217

FIG. 218

FIG. 214

FIG. 219

FIG. 215

FIG. 220

FIG. 212 and FIG. 216.—The patient has five devitalized teeth with granulomata. One tooth had to be extracted on each side. The treatment. filling. bridgework and apicectomy which was finally performed is seen in Figs. 213, 214 and 215, for one side, Figs. 217, 218, 219 and 220 for the other side.

the eyes, nose, and mouth. It goes without saying that the operator wears sterile gowns and gloves.

Operation. The saliva ejector is put in place by the assistant and the lip is retracted with a lip retractor. One sterile syringe is placed on either side of the part that is to be operated so as to prevent saliva entering the field of operation. The mucous membrane is dried with sterile gauze and painted with $3\frac{1}{2}$ per cent. iodine or aqueous solution of iodine.

Incision. With a flap knife make a "U"-shaped incision, as shown in the picture. Lift the periosteum and gum from the bone with the sharp periosteal elevator. Insert a suitable gum retractor and use sterile gauze to remove the blood.

Amputation of the Root. The alveolar process is now visible if it has not been destroyed by the granulation. A good-sized opening is cut with the chisel and mallet, or by aid of the burr to get a clear view of the apex of the root. Resect the apex with a fissure burr at a point further down than the extent of the root-canal filling and as far toward the cervical part as is necessary to remove all parts which are necrosed. Remove the resected apex with a suitable elevator.

Curetting of the Abscess Cavity. The most important part is still ahead. This is the removal of the granulation tissue and curetting of the alveolar process with a round burr, until all granulation and osteomyelitic bone is removed and healthy bone is visible on all sides.

Treatment of the Wound. Smooth carefully with the burr all sharp points and margins of the alveolar process. Do not shape the distal part of the tooth like the end of a root, as it is sometimes advised, because this still decreases the amount of attachment with the bone. Also, I prefer to have one round, clean cavity without anything projecting into it. Wash with normal salt solution, remove all the débris, sponge, and sterilize the whole cavity with $3\frac{1}{2}$ per cent. iodine or aqueous solution of iodine. Remove the excess with sterile sponges and stimulate bleeding with a suitable instrument. When the cavity is filled up with a blood clot, draw the flap over the opening and sew it carefully with three horse hair stitches.

Healing. If proper aseptic care has been taken, a good union of the gum is obtained in a short time. The stitches are removed after three days and if horsehair has been used, this causes little or no discomfort. In my mind, the sewing in the mouth is of greatest importance; it prevents reinfection from saliva and the fluids of the mouth. The healing of the bone cavity occurs by organization of the blood clot, and bone is later formed from this tissue. In some of the radiographs it can be seen how the trabeculae of bone grow into the cavity. Ultimately the tooth becomes ankylosed at the end to the newly-formed bone. The patient should be told that the face may swell up the following day as a result of the mechanical injury, for which dry heat can be applied. After three or four days the face is normal again. After-pain is very seldom noticed.

Failures and Dangers.

The anatomical relations of the jaw should be kept in mind: in the upper jaw the proximity of the antrum, in the lower bicuspid region the mental foramen, and if operating on the lower molars the relation to the mandibular canal. If the operation is performed with perfect aseptic precautions there is very little danger. Failures, however, may occur either because the granulation tissue has not been entirely removed, because a neighboring tooth may be involved, because the tooth has not been sterilized, or because the cement of the root may be discolored and necrotic almost to the cervical margin. The last two reasons are the most important ones and always cause reinfection, which can only be cured by extraction. I want to make it very plain that this operation is not a short cut to save the removal of a crown, and proper treatment of the root canal, and it is only successful if that work has been previously accomplished satisfactorily.

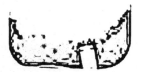

Fig. 222

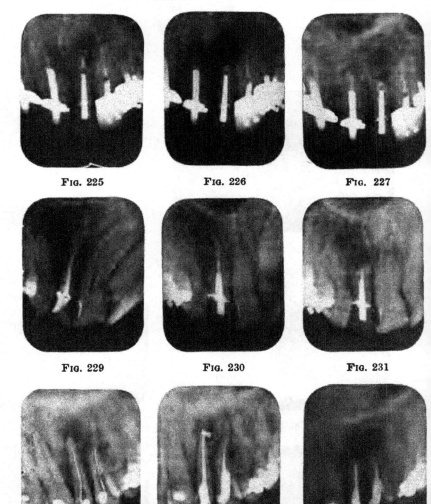

Fig. 222

Fig. 223

Fig. 225

Fig. 226

Fig. 227

Fig. 229

Fig. 230

Fig. 231

Fig. 232

Fig. 233

Fig. 234

Fig. 235

221, 222, 223, 224, 225, 226 and 227.—Radiographs showing the different steps of root canal treatment an
my on a lateral incisor, which had imperfect root filling and apical granuloma. Fig. 226, taken directly afte
operation. Fig. 227 four months later.

28, 229, 230 and 231.—Radiographs showing the treatment for apiectomy on another lateral incisor. Fig. 231 i
wo months after the operation, the bone is starting to fill in. The excised granuloma of this case is seen in Figs
134 and 135.

32, 233, 234 and 235.—Radiographs showing the process of apiectomy on two teeth, the lateral incisor and cuspid

PLATE LXVIII

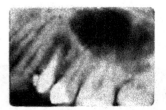

FIG. 236

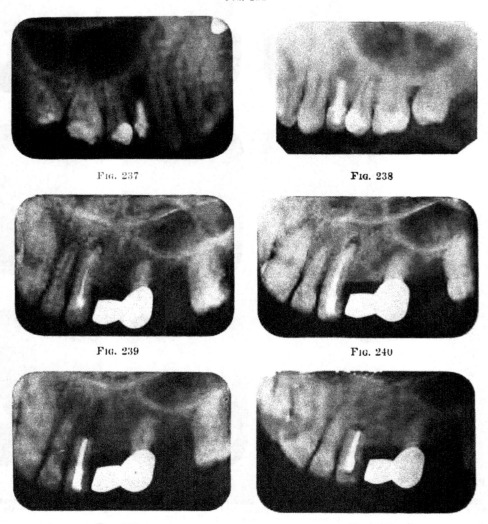

FIG. 237

FIG. 238

FIG. 239

FIG. 240

FIG. 241

FIG. 242

FIGS. 236, 237 and 238.—Radiographs showing apiectomy on a first bicuspid. Fig. 23 immediately after the operation. Fig. 238 shows the process of healing, six months later.

FIGS. 239, 240, 241 and 242.—Apiectomy on a cuspid. Fig. 241 directly after the operation. Fig. 242, nine months after the operation.

EXTRACTION AND CURETTAGE If apiectomy is ruled out as the advisable treatment for one reason or another, we still have the most radical treatment left; this is extraction of the tooth and curettage of the bone. This treatment radically and positively removes not only the lesion, but also its cause. I lay great stress on the removal of the chronic abscess with the curette or surgical burr. After washing the wound, the alveolar socket should be inspected and curetting is repeated if all has not been removed. Very frequently we find a definite abscess in the radiograph, but after the tooth has been extracted, there is no abscess attached to the tooth, and if we inspect the socket there is only bone to be seen. This may be due to the fact that the lamella of the alveolar socket has not been destroyed by the disease and that it has to be broken through at the bottom if we want to reach the granulation. After the curetting has been completed the wound is again inspected, and if all the bone looks healthy, I sterilize the wound with $3\frac{1}{2}\%$ iodine or aqueous solution of iodine, and then allow the socket to fill with blood. The blood clot will organize and form new tissue.

After the bleeding is stopped, the patient is instructed to use a mouth wash, and is asked to return for inspection of the healing wound and for treatment.

In severe systemic disorders, if the patient has a low resistance, or in any weak person, it is necessary to use proper judgment in determining the number of teeth that are to be extracted at one time. I have in many cases ·noticed an exacerbation after surgical treatment, and Hartzel reports that he has noted an exacerbation of joint inflammation in all arthritic patients following surgical treatment of pyorrhoea or curettage of abscesses. A sudden extensive removal of a large number of lesions may cause positive harm, especially in weakened patients who have suffered a long time, and where the protective cells have been worn out from long-continued chronic focal infection. It is therefore not advisable to extract a large number of teeth at one sitting, or to remove all the teeth and the tonsils the same day, while the successive removal of the foci will benefit the patient; the action of this process will be described later under surgical auto-inoculation.

EXTIRPATION OF TEETH The extirpation of teeth with chisel or burr, or both, is an operation performed as the last resort, if extraction by forceps and elevator have failed. But often it is indicated as a typical primary operation, if the case is diagnosed as a difficult one by means of radiographic examination.

Indication. Extirpation of roots and teeth is specially indicated in cases of extensive exostosis of the root apices, or in cases of broken down roots, partly or entirely covered by the gum, and especially if the distal teeth have moved forward so that the root is too large for the space.

Anaesthesia. Local anaesthesia or local and general anaesthesia combined can be used. The decreased bleeding obtained by local injections is desirable, especially in the back of the mouth.

Preparation. Sensitive and apprehensive patients should receive a sedative, such as Bromural-Knoll, two tablets to adults, in water, thirty minutes before the operation, if local anaesthesia is used. One hour before the operation ¼ gram of morphia with or without atropin, as required, hypodermically, is used before a general anaesthetic.

Preparing the Field of Operation. The mucous membrane should be dried and the area to be operated on is painted with tincture of iodine or aqueous solution of iodine. The saliva is taken care of by the saliva ejector.

Incision. Several types of incisions are used according to location and condition. It should be large enough to prevent laceration of the soft tissue and give a clear view of the field of operation.

Operation. After the retractors are inserted remove the outer part of the alveolar process, so as to expose the entire root or roots; in molars the roots should next be separated, and this is best done with a fissure burr. The root or roots are then luxated with an elevator, after which the sockets are curetted and the edges of the bone

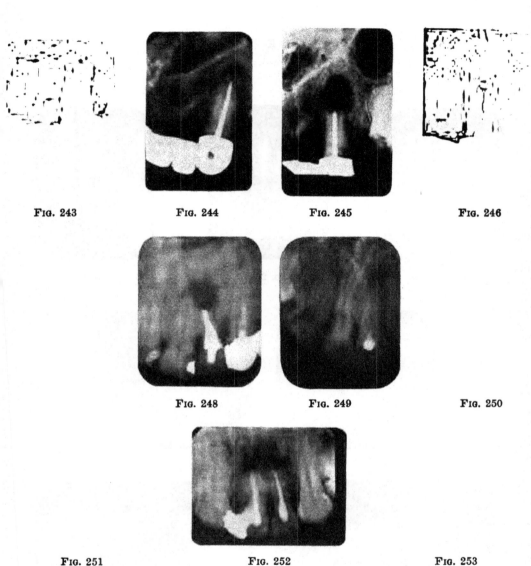

FIG. 243   FIG. 244   FIG. 245   FIG. 246

FIG. 248   FIG. 249   FIG. 250

FIG. 251   FIG. 252   FIG. 253

FIGS. 243, 244, 245 and 246.—Apiectomy on a cuspid which is an abutment for a bridge. The pulp had died. No root filling. Fig. 244 shows root filling. Fig. 245, immediately after the operation. Fig. 246, after eight months.

FIGS. 247 and 248.—Apiectomy on a lateral incisor.

FIGS. 249 and 250.—Apiectomy on a central incisor.

FIGS. 251, 252 and 253.—Apiectomy on two teeth, central and lateral incisors. Fig. 251, directly after the operation. Fig. 252 shows the healing process after two months. Fig. 253 shows the bone completely filled in after ten months.

PLATE LXX

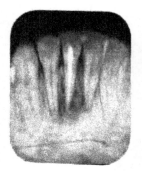
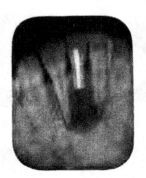
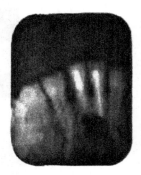

FIG. 254   FIG. 255   FIG. 256

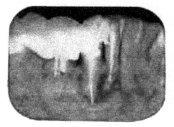
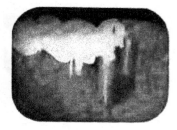

FIG. 257   FIG. 258

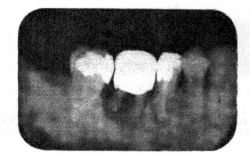
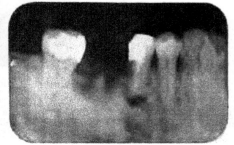

FIG. 259   FIG. 260

FIGS. 254 and 255.—Apiectomy on a lower incisor.

FIG. 256.—Apiectomy on two lower incisors.

FIGS. 257 and 258.—Apiectomy on a lower incisor with broken root instrument in apical part of the root canal.

FIGS. 259 and 260.—Apiectomy on a lower bicuspid, the molar was extracted at the same sitting.

smoothed with the surgical burr. It is important to remove all pieces of process which are fractured or projecting so as not to prolong or hinder the healing process.

Care of Wound. The gum should be placed back and sutured to its original position. The wound is washed with normal salt solution until all débris is removed, and then treated with 3½ per cent. tincture of iodine or aqueous solution of iodine. In cases of chronic abscesses the wound can be filled in with a blood clot if the curettage has been performed properly, but in cases of active suppuration, I prefer to pack the socket with iodoform gauze, saturated with orthoform or novocain powder to prevent pain. A mixture of orthoform powder, novocain, and campho-phenique is also most excellent for this purpose. The wound should be irrigated and dressed until filled in with granulations.

3. *Treatment of Abscesses Due to Diseases of the Gum.*

Abscesses Due to Injury of the Gum. The abscesses which start at the gingival part of the gum respond easily to treatment as soon as the cause is removed. Foreign substances, irritating fillings or crowns should be taken care of, the abscesses should be incised and washed out. Iodine is most effective as a therapeutic agent.

Abscesses Due to Pus Pockets. Abscesses caused by the closing of a pyorrhoea pocket should be incised to evacuate the pus. The tooth is scaled until all débris attached to it are removed. After washing with normal salt solution, treatment with iodine is found beneficial. Ionic treatment is also highly recommended. Most of these cases are due to pyorrhoea and the treatment of pyorrhoea will not be considered in this book.

4. *Treatment of Abscesses Due to Difficult Eruption, Impaction and Unerupted Teeth.*

Radiographic examination is imperative in all cases of impacted and unerupted teeth, not only to make sure of the diagnosis, but also to find out the position of the tooth and to determine the course of treatment. Intraoral films often give good results, but generally I prefer a plate. With many patients it is hard to use an intraoral film on account of trismus or a sensitive throat, and often we get only the crown of the tooth in the picture, and while it is possible to determine from this how the crown is interlocked, it leaves us in doubt about the formation of the roots. From this radiograph we should be able to ascertain the number of roots, their form, as well as the location of the tooth in regard to the ramus and mandibular canal.

EXTIRPATION OF IMPACTED AND UNERUPTED TEETH All impacted teeth which give rise to pathological conditions, such as abscess pockets or pain caused by pressure, neural and mental irritation, should be promptly extirpated. This involves a difficult and serious operation in which sometimes the skill of the oral surgeon is taxed to its highest degree. The technique of the operation I shall not mention here, but a few words about pre-anaesthetic medication, anaesthesia and after-treatment may be of use. The physician has not yet generally appreciated the difficulty of this operation, and the dentist has not until lately recognized the value of proper preparation and the after-treatment necessary for the extirpation of impacted teeth, as well as other oral surgical operations. If the operation is performed under local conductive anaesthesia, which is the anaesthesia of choice, it should be preceded by administration of an hypnotic or narcotic, such as Bromural-Knoll, two tablets in water half an hour before the operation, or in more serious cases, morphine gr. 1/6 to gr. 1/4, or morphine, gr. 1/4, and atropine, gr. 1/150. This stupifies the patient so as to take away the terror of the operation, and apprehension of the instrumentation. It also relieves the after-pain associated with such an operation. Many patients, however, prefer a general anaesthetic, which also should be preceded by the usual preanaesthetic medication. General and local anaesthesia may be combined to great advantage to overcome the physical as well as psychic shock. All depends of course a good deal upon the attitude of the patient and the difficulty of the case. A good many impacted or unerupted teeth can be extir-

PLATE LXXI

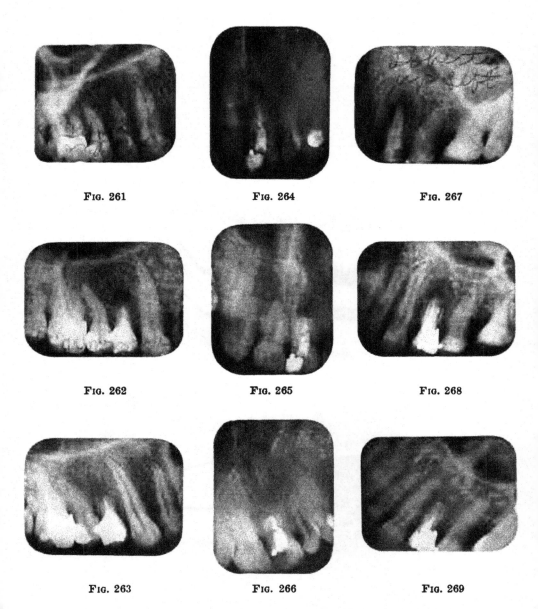

FIG. 261

FIG. 264

FIG. 267

FIG. 262

FIG. 265

FIG. 268

FIG. 263

FIG. 266

FIG. 269

FIGS. 261, 262 and 263.—Series of radiographs showing healing of the bone cavity. Fig. 262, immediately after operation. Fig. 263, after about one year.

FIGS. 264, 265 and 266.—The condition before the operation is seen in Fig. 264. Fig. 265 shows the healing after a few weeks. Fig. 266 shows complete filling in of the bone cavity after about fourteen months.

FIGS. 267, 268, 269.—Radiographs showing the healing process after apiectomy. Fig. 268 shows bridges of bone growing into the cavity. Fig. 269 the condition after about one year.

PLATE LXXII

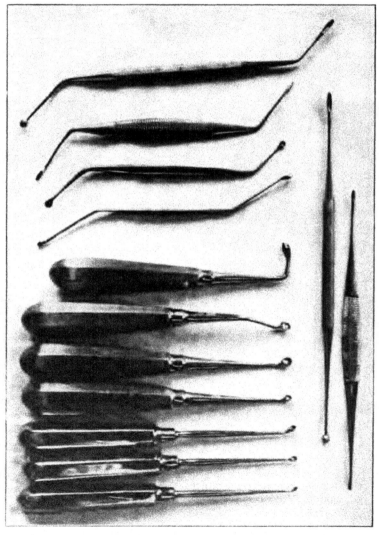

FIG. 270.—A selection of curettes.

pated without great effort, and in a comparatively short time, while others call into action the greatest operating skill. The easy cases can easily be performed in the office, while hard cases, in apprehensive and neurasthenic patients, should be done at the hospital, where the patient can receive proper preanaesthetic treatment and have proper care and medication for a few days. After the operation great pain is usually experienced, especially after the removal of lower impacted wisdom teeth, which frequently extend into the mandibular canal. To combat the pain, give morphia gr. 1/6 to gr. ¼ hypodermically, later, if the pain is less severe, the following powders have been found excellent by the author:

℞

Phenacetin	....	0.7	gr. xii
Sodium bicarbonate	......	1.03	gr. xx
Codeine sulphate	....	0.06	gr. i
Caffeine citrate	....	0.24	gr. iv

Mx et devide chartulas in powders No2 iv.
Sig. One powder every three hours until relieved.

If there is only a small amount of pain prescribe:

Phenacetin—
Aspirin ......aa.   2.0   gr. xxx

Mx et devide chartulas in powders No2 vi.
Sig. Take one powder every hour until relieved.

5. *Treatment of Abscesses of the Tongue.*

The treatment of abscesses of the tongue depends very much upon the duration of the lesion and the differentiation of the simple, the phlegmonous, and tubercular type.

INCISION IN NONTUBERCULAR LESIONS

In simple abscesses of the tongue with only moderate infiltration, a small deep incision is all that is necessary. The abscess cavity is drained and kept open by an iodoform wicking, which is changed until suppuration has stopped and the wound healed. In the severe type of phlegmonous abscess of the tongue, it is important to incise as early as possible. General anaesthesia is usually necessary to open the mouth, which is locked by muscular trismus, so that the tongue can be properly palpitated and the cause ascertained. The anaesthetic should be given by a method which makes aspiration of pus and blood impossible. If an abscess is the cause of the disease, this should be widely opened first, and if due to a tooth or teeth, these should be extracted without hesitation. The tongue then is drawn forwards and pressed towards the healthy side. Its muscle is deeply incised with a crescent-shaped knife by a horizontal cut, which should start as far back as possible and reach way forward near the point through the thick, ungainly, deformed substance of the tongue. There may be not much discharge of pus from the tongue, except a small amount of badly smelling liquid, which almost always flows from the wound. This is, however, enough to lessen the dangerous increase of the swelling and give relief to the angina, feared more than anything else by the patient. The mouth gag should stay in the mouth until the patient has awakened, when the danger of aspiring blood and pus is passed.

EXCISION OF SMALL TUBERCULAR LESIONS   Small tubercular lesions should be thoroughly excised and the wound sutured immediately. Lactic acid is used by Brophy to sterilize the wound, and the use of the X-rays is recommended as postoperative treatment.

V-SHAPED EXCISION OF THE TONGUE   This operation is recommended by Krause and Heymann for tuberculosis, gumma, benign tumors and selected malignant tumors which involve only the tip of the tongue. Under anaesthesia the tongue is drawn forward and a thread of heavy silk is then drawn through each side as far back as possible. These hold the tongue in position. A V-shaped incision is now made in the healthy tissue, a good distance away from the diseased part. In order to lose the least amount of blood, the incision is only made two-

PLATE LXXIII

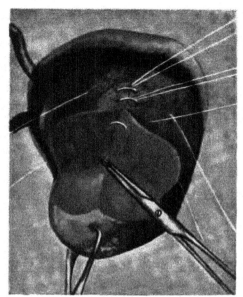

FIG. 271

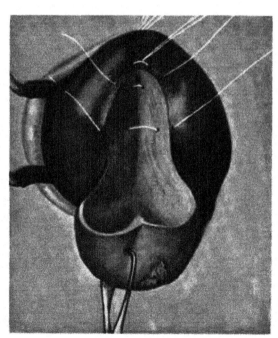

FIG. 272

FIGS. 271 and 272.—Excision of tip of tongue as
described in text.

thirds deep, the anterior part is held with a tongue forceps and drawn forward, and silk sutures are inserted at once to draw the two sides together. After several stitches are inserted, the incision is continued towards the floor of the mouth on one side. When the lingual artery is divided, the vessel should be seized with a haemostatic forceps and ligated. The same thing is done on the other side. The sutures are continued while the two sides are drawn together. A new tip is thus formed by the dorsal part of the tongue; this is drawn up so that the lower surface becomes accessible. The diseased part of the tongue is now hanging down and the suturing is continued while the tip is resected, bringing the surfaces in exact contact. Finally the excised part is severed and the remaining wound united. The two large pieces of silk which served to draw the tongue forward are removed, but two of the threads from the sutures are left and fastened, one on each cheek, to pull the tongue forward in case of post-operative oedema. Liquid diet should be prescribed, which is to be given through a glass tube.

Large tubercular abscesses of the tongue, especially those on the side and extending down to the reflection of the mucous membrane of the floor of the mouth, cannot be operated upon as just described. These should be curetted. Brophy recommends application of lactic acid and the X-ray. He says that the results of treatment of tuberculosis of the tongue are not gratifying, and that this is primarily due to the fact that the patient is much debilitated by the presence of tuberculosis in other parts of the body, therefore one should be guarded in his prognosis.

6. Treatment of Abscesses of the Salivary Glands and Ducts.

Abscesses of salivary glands and ducts are almost always associated with salivary calculi, which are ascertained and diagnosed by means of radiographs. Surgical interference therefore is always necessary.

Abscesses and calculi, which are formed in the glandular ducts, can almost always be excised from the inside of the mouth, except in Wharton's duct, which we can only trace as far back as the myohyoid muscle from this region. Also the sublingual gland is accessible from the inside of the mouth, while the submaxillary gland, however, and the posterior part of its duct, as well as the parotid gland, can only be reached by an incision through the skin.

OPERATION FROM THE FLOOR OF THE MOUTH After the mouth has been opened under ether the tongue is seized with a pair of tongue forceps and drawn towards the corner of the mouth on the healthy side, the lower part turned up. The tongue now can be retracted so that we get good access to the field of operation. Pack the pharynx with gauze and apply iodine for sterilization. An incision is made halfway between the frenum of the tongue and the inner surface of the jaw, and parallel with the latter. The mucous membrane is carefully dissected away and retracted. Part of Wharton's duct is now visible, and if it harbors the stone it should be dissected (lingual nerve towards the mesial side). Split the duct lengthwise directly over the stone. This is then removed, after which a fine probe may be inserted through the ranuncula salivaris, over which the opening of the duct can be closed with a few sutures. If the stone, however, is not found to be in this duct, or if it had been diagnosed from the beginning to be in the sublingual gland, we should first ascertain its exact location by puncturing the gland with a straight and fine steel needle. If we draw pus or feel hard resistance we know that we are near. The way to the stone should be secured by a blunt instrument injuring as little of the glandular substance as possible. A fine haemostatic forceps serves well for taking hold of the stone, and after it is removed the pus should be washed out with salt solution, tincture of iodine may be applied, after which the mucous membrane is closed by catgut sutures. In the experience of the author great relief and speedy improvement follows this operation.

EXCISION OF THE GLANDS In cases where the stone cannot be removed from the inside of the mouth, excision of the whole gland is advisable to prevent salivary fistulas. The same is true in cases of extensive destruction of any of the glands. If a fistula exists already it is sometimes due to obstruction in the excretory duct, the relief of which has been found to cause speedy healing of the fistula.

7. *Treatment of Systemic Complications.*

The important factor in treatment of systemic complications is the early removal of the focus. If foci have been in an active state for a considerable period of time the disease becomes firmly fixed, the secondary infection may be well established, and in the persistent stage tissue destruction may have occurred; this condition is beyond repair. Elimination of the focus then does little in the way of repair, although it prevents reinfection and removes a septic condition which is a great burden to the system, wearing out the organs, the duty of which is to protect the body by destroying the bacteria and neutralizing the foreign ferments and protein poisons.

If a result is expected from the removal of the focus of a disease, it is of utmost importance not only to find and remove the primary focus, but also others, namely, the secondary foci caused by hematogenesis from the primary focus, as these are new factors which will continue the trouble. A streptococcus infection of the tonsils may, for example, have been the primary cause of an endocarditis or acute arthritis, but they also may have produced a streptococcus infection in two chronic alveolar granulomata which heretofore had been caused by staphylococci albi. After the removal of the tonsils, the infection continues from the streptococcus infection of the dental granulomata and we fail to get a cure. No time therefore should be lost in acute hopeful conditions to ascertain all foci, whether primary or secondary, and promptly start in with their radical removal.

SURGICAL AUTO-INOC-ULATION This, however, should be undertaken in a systematic way, and not as one multiple operation, as such procedure could, under certain circumstances as we have seen, bring positive harm. The surgical interference necessarily inoculates the patient with a large number of organisms, inducing an effect similar to that of an efficient vaccine, with the added advantage that the constant supply is shut off from the disturbed focus. This surgical auto-inoculation stimulates the production of antibodies benefiting the patient after each operation, bringing about a gradual gain. It can readily be seen that a too large inoculation would cause positive harm, especially in a patient who is weakened and has lost his resistance by long standing disease. The removal of the foci should, therefore, be carefully planned; three to six days should elapse between each operation. Not only should foci in different parts of the body be removed at different times, but also foci in one region should, if possible, be operated on with intermission. In the mouth, for example, abscessed teeth should be extracted and curetted one at a time, leaving three to six days between each operation, and here again I want to impress the importance of thorough curettage, because it not only removes the principal part, the real focus, which otherwise may continue to feed the infection, but also surgical auto-inoculation is wholly dependent upon thorough disturbance of the focus.

In most diseases treatment of the secondary manifestations is to be undertaken hand in hand with the removal of the focus, because we can not expect that pathological changes in the new lesions disappear without the proper care and attention. Medical therapeutics, massage, hydrotherapeutics, surgical interference, rest, or exercise, fresh air, cheerful surroundings, regulation of diet and improvement in digestion and assimilation, all will further improvement and cure of the disease.

RESTORATION OF MASTICATING EFFICIENCY One of the factors which improves the patient's digestive process, and with it his health and strength, is proper mastication of the food. We cannot expect that the stomach of a weakened patient, whom we desire to build up, will digest food which has not been properly prepared in the mouth. It is therefore of greatest importance to replace all teeth, those which have been previously lost and those which had to be sacrificed to get rid of a primary or secondary infectious focus. The mouth should as soon as possible be restored to its full and important physiologic action by plates or removable bridge work.

CHAPTER XI

PREVENTION

Gigantic studies have been made both in medicine and dentistry in the last twenty or thirty years. The most important advances, perhaps, are those of preventive medicine and hygiene, and from all the specialties of medicine there is none in which prevention is more important than in dentistry. Disease of a tooth means invariably loss of substance; whether it is hard or soft tissue, restoration to normal is seldom possible, a decayed tooth will never fill in, an inflamed pulp will not yield to any treatment, and the result is always loss of part of the tooth or of the whole organ. The treatment is a replacement of the lost organic substance by inorganic material, metal or porcelain, and the result is a compromise of a more or less temporary character.

The importance of the oral hygiene movement has been acknowledged by the physician, the schools, and the public, and it is general knowledge that teeth should be saved for masticating purposes and that insufficient mastication, from lack of teeth, often causes malnutrition. Today, however, there is connected with oral hygiene a still greater factor than saving teeth for mastication; this is prevention of septic conditions in the mouth. We have seen that the mouth is the very gateway through which disease may enter and proceed through various channels to almost any part of the body. In our practical hospitals and clinics we have occasion to see patients where disease is well on the way, so that it is too late for a cure of the secondary chronic disease; we see a large number of patients where we can stop disease by removing the septic condition, and in still others we shall be able to prevent septic oral foci by judiciously selecting favorable cases only for root canal treatment, advising extraction of those teeth which cannot properly be taken care of. Our greatest effort, however, should be directed towards educating the public to make them realize the importance of preserving the vitality of the tooth and prevent decay, which is almost always the primary cause of pulp disease and dental abscesses. The gums should be kept in healthy condition so as to prevent pyorrhoea, which is a disease of almost equal frequency.

Prevention of Secondary Diseases from Oral Abscesses.

At another place we have discussed the privilege and duty of the dentist to participate in the diagnosis of the cause of secondary disease and the aid in treatment, by judiciously and radically removing such foci, if abscesses or other septic conditions are found in the mouth. The difficulty in obtaining a speedy cure by the removal of the focus after the secondary disease has passed into a chronic stage, has been pointed out at various places, and the advantage of removing such foci for prevention is therefore obvious. Each individual mouth should be examined most carefully by means of instrumentation and radiographs, and all septic conditions should be radically removed. If it seems advisable to treat these teeth in a conservative way by carefully sterilizing and filling the root canals, subsequent examination by the radiograph at regular intervals is indicated to note whether there is improvement or whether the condition is getting worse. It may be hard for a man who has practised for years the saving of every tooth at any cost, to make up his mind to advise extraction or expensive root-canal treatment if there is no apparent local trouble in the mouth, and it will be hard for a patient to understand why this or that tooth which does not ache, could be a factor of present or future ill-health, and should be treated or removed, unless the dentist is able to explain the condition in a convincing manner, which can only be based upon a thorough understanding of the condition. But he who does not tolerate septic conditions in his patient's mouth practises good dentistry as far as the teeth are concerned, and most excellent preventive medicine from the standpoint of the whole body.

Prevention of Periapical Infection.

The question whether or not abscesses on devitalized teeth can be prevented has not yet been entirely solved. The men (Ulrich*) who believe that these abscesses are caused principally by haematogenous infections of the periapical area of pulpless teeth, which represents tissue of lower resistance, think that it does not matter how well the root canals are filled, abscesses may be caused in any case, if there are infectious foci in other parts of the body, which cause a mild bacteremia. They claim that it is especially the streptococcus to which the lesion may be attributed and look at most apical abscesses as secondary infections. However, we need not search for very remote modes of infection when there are other causes nearer at hand. If we consider the anatomy and pathology of the dental pulp, if we remember how hard it is to render aseptic the root canal, the dentinal tubules and the apical foramina, and how often careless methods of technique are employed, we find the causes may be practically obvious. However, I do not doubt that in some instances abscesses start as a secondary infection, and furthermore, that subacute attacks of abscesses which have been in the quiescent stage of inflammation for many years may perhaps be explained in this way, although here again we have other factors to consider.

RADIO-GRAPHIC DIAGNOSIS BEFORE ROOT CANAL TREATMENT It is well to radiograph a tooth before undertaking to treat a root canal, no matter what condition it is in. Abnormal formation of the   s and obstructions such as deposits of secondary dentine and pulpstones can in this way be determined beforehand, and the patient and the dentist save much time and expense if it is determined, whether or not we can mechanically achieve a perfect result.

* ULRICH, HENRY L.: The Blind Abscess. *Journal of the American Medical Association*, November 6, 1915, p. 1619.

PLATE LXXIV

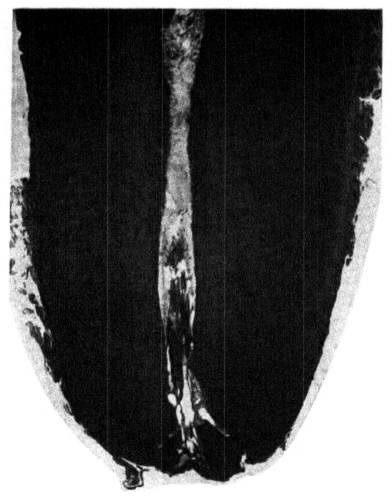

FIG. 273.—Microphotograph of the apex of a tooth showing multiple
foramina.

*Specimen by author and stained with Mallory's Phosphotungstic
acid and Hematoxylin.*

ANAESTHESIA FOR PULP EXTIRPATION Grieves* points out that arsenic used for devitalization of a pulp is very apt to cause necrosis in the periapical tissue on account of its vascularity, the drug being absorbed by the pulp. Pressure anaesthesia with novocain or cocaine as first described by Professor Edward C. Briggs of Boston, is of greatest value for pulp extirpation. Local anaesthesia with novocain suprarenin† is also very excellent, and many times the only method that gives results, as in cases of diseased pulps with persisting nerve fibres or partly extirpated pulps. General anaesthesia is not recommended except in front teeth where the procedure is comparatively simple.

COMPLETE PULP EXTIRPATION If a pulp is infected or disturbed by surgical interference, it strangles itself at the apical foramen on account of the hyperemia produced. It is therefore important to remove every particle of it, or later it will become a source for periapical infection.

In pulp extirpation a fine broach should be inserted as far into the root canal as possible so that the entire pulp is removed at once. A fine wire with a loop should then be inserted with the mild antiseptic dressing, and another radiograph should be taken to find out whether we have reached the end of the root.

CLEANING AND ENLARGING THE CANAL If the root canal is not large enough to allow easy passage to its end, and if diseased or healthy tissue remains, this should be taken care of by the sulphuric acid or sodium potassum method. Both of these drugs are valuable for root canal work, but care should be taken not to force any through the apical foramen. The sulphuric acid should be neutralized with sodium bicarbonate; both drugs are best used in Luer syringes with root canal hub. The sodium potassium paste is used on smooth broaches; its great affinity for organic matter draws the drug through obstructed places,

* GRIEVES, CLARENCE J.: *Dental Cosmos*, October, 1915, p. 1118.
† THOMA, KURT H.: Oral Anaesthesia, p. 107.

making passage way for the broach. The result, however, depends a great deal upon patient and continued instrumentation. The Rhein picks are the most valuable instruments for this purpose. The strong caustic alkali which is formed by this process should be neutralized by sulphuric acid, and this in turn by sodium bicarbonate. An important factor in root canal operations is easy access, for the crown of the tooth should be so reduced as to allow straight entrance into the canals.

ANTISEPTIC MEDICATION Failure of achieving the desired results in root-canal operations has gradually led to the use of highly oxidizing, tissue obstructing drugs with great penetrating power, in the age when older antiseptic methods have almost entirely yielded to good surgery, and where it is an important principal to destroy as few cells as possible, and where we know that any cell which is rendered necrotic adds only another place where infection may find media of its liking. Drugs, such as formaldehyde and all its numerous preparations, should not be placed into a *root canal* under any condition. Formaldehyde preparations should only be used as the first dressing upon a putrescent pulp, placed into *the pulp chamber,* and covered with cotton saturated in petrol oil or with temporary stopping, as the case requires. After the pulp has been extirpated, this drug should no longer be applied into the pulp chamber nor into the root canal, as it would penetrate through the foramen and do harm to the periapical tissue. Zinc chloride, copper sulphate, concentrated phenol, trichloracetic acid are other root-canal drugs of great tissue destroying action. Their use as well as the use of sulphuric acid and sodium potassium for root-canal cleaning should be carefully controlled, and great care should be taken to confine their action to the root canal. G. V. Black* describes at length experiments made by application of the different drugs for use in root canal treatment. The different medicaments were applied to the skin on cotton in small rubber cups, held in position by

* BLACK, G. V.: Special Dental Pathology, pp. 291-298.

Fig. 274.—Microphotograph of the end of a root.

A, showing root filling extending into a remnant of pulp which
may give a symptom of pain which often is mistaken for the
pain caused when emerging through the apical foramen.
B, Necrosed area of the dentine. D, Pulp remnant.
C, Secondary dentine filling the canal.

*Specimen prepared by the author. Stained by Mallory's
Phosphotungstic acid and Hematoxylin.*

court plaster. Oil of cloves and Blackwood creosote each produced practically no inflammation, Black's 1, 2, 3 only slight irritation, oil of cinnamon a large blister, creosol and formalin in each instance a very deep inflammation which was painful and so unbearable that it had to be removed after seven hours; the tissue formed no blister but was of yellowish color as though it would slough away; needles could be stuck into the tissue one-third of an inch before sensation was felt. Six weeks later a scar was visible which looked as though the area had been burned. It is evident that such an injurious drug should not be sealed into root canals.

To avoid injury of the periodontal membrane and bone surrounding the apex of the tooth, the operator should put his effort into perfecting his technique rather than relying on strong drugs to sterilize what he neglected to remove. Mild antiseptics and anodines are sufficient as dressings in most cases, ionic application of iodine will take care of bacteria in dentinal tubules and accessory foramina, and if a healthy condition cannot be obtained by mild medication, the cause is to be looked for outside the tooth. If a radiograph was not taken beforehand, it is now time to find out the condition of the periapical tissue, and in most cases it will be found that the reason of not making any headway is due to a granuloma or chronic abscess, a lesion which does not yield to medicinal treatment. Mild antiseptics of reputation are:

Black's 1, 2, 3.

℞

    Ol. cassiae ....1 part
    Thenolis ....2 parts
    Ol. Gaulteriae ....3 parts
Mx the oils and add melted crystals of phenol.

Buckley's Modified Phenol.

℞

    Mentholis ....gr. xx
    Thymolis ....gr. xl
    Phenolis ....f3 iii

IONIC MEDICATION Ionic medication has already been considered for treatment of periodontitis. Zinc chloride and copper sulphate should not be used for sterilization of dental structures on account of their tissue destroying action, upon which some men base the treatment of the apical granuloma. This is believed to be dissolved by this method so that it can be resorbed by the tissue. Such applications, however, also destroy the periodontal membrane, and as we have seen that the success of root canal treatment depends upon preservation of this most important structure, it would be unwise to apply an agent which has exactly the opposite effect.

Iodine ions are, however, to be recommended for root canal or rather dentine sterilization. Tincture of iodine $3\frac{1}{2}$ per cent. or aqueous solution of iodine, a recent preparation without the irritating action of the alcohol, is applied into the root canal by means of a Luer syringe. The negative pole is applied to a platinum broach, with cotton saturated in the same solution attached, the positive pole is placed under the rubber dam in the form of a sponge electrode, or held in the hand. The circuit of a direct current, reduced by a special rheostat (there are several well made ionization machines in the market) and measured by a milliampere meter is now closed and the amount is gradually increased until from $\frac{1}{2}$ to 3 milliampere is used. The treatment should be applied for ten minutes in each canal. Iodine should be added from time to time, as it is used up quickly, which is indicated by the white color of the peripheral part of the dressing. After ionic medication with iodine the pulp chamber should be washed out with alcohol or acetone to remove the brown stain. A mild aseptic dressing is inserted and the canals filled at another sitting.

The most important factor which has to do with poor root-canal filling and following periapical infection is unsuccessful dehydration. Acetone should be applied by means of Luer syringe and broach, and dried out with hot compressed air. An electric root-canal dryer is then

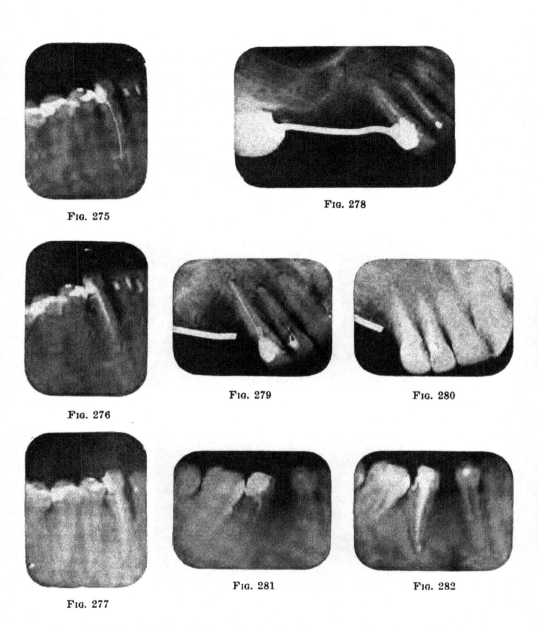

FIG. 275

FIG. 278

FIG. 276

FIG. 279

FIG. 280

FIG. 277

FIG. 281

FIG. 282

FIGS. 275, 276 and 277.—Radiographs showing the process of root canal treatment.
Fig. 275, shows a wire which was inserted to see whether the apex was reached.
Fig. 276 shows an unsuccessful root canal filling.   Fig. 277 the final filling.
FIGS. 278, 279 and 280.—Radiograph No. 278, showing two teeth not filled to the end.
Fig. 279, radiographs with wires inserted.   Fig. 280 shows the canal fillings.
FIGS. 281, 282.   Radiograph No. 281 shows ''corkscrew'' filling which was replaced
by filling seen in Fig. 282.

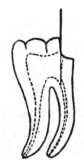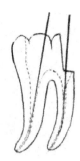

FIG. 283

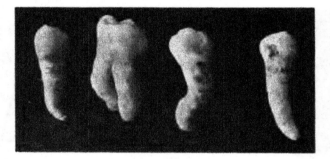

FIG. 284

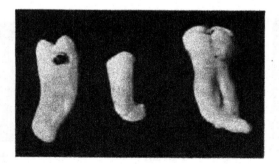

FIG. 285

FIG. 285.—On left root treatment attempted through small cavity, the broach does not go around the curve. On right mesio-occlusial cavity cut extensively, so as to get proper access to canals.

FIG. 284 and 285.—Specimen of bent and curved roots, the root canals of which would be hard to treat and fill.

inserted and if used for the first time the operator will be surprised to hear a sizzling noise, indicating that there was still some moisture left. The heat is applied until the patient feels the warmth. For root-canal filling the author prefers the chloroform-resin-gutta-percha method.* The chloroform and resin (d.i to gr. iv) is best applied into the canal by use of an ordinary Luer Q syringe; with a smooth broach carefully remove all air bubbles. Select a sterile gutta-percha cone or point and pump it into the canal forty times. The chloroform dissolves the gutta percha, which is forced into the fine canals and foramina by the pumping action. Other cones follow the first until the canal is filled, when the filling is condensed with a root canal condenser. This method has several advantages; the most important ones are that newly-formed chloro-percha can be forced into the finest canals without the evaporation which spoils the result in other methods, and that the excess forced through the foramina is not a sharp point projecting into the peri-apical tissue, but a soft paste which caps the apex, so to speak, adapting itself on its surface. A radiograph is taken immediately, and in case the filling does not reach to the apex it can be removed before it has hardened, when the same process is repeated until the filling is satisfactory.

STERILIZA-TION AND ASEPSIS Sterilization of the instruments and aseptic methods cannot be too strongly insisted upon. If we consider that the bacteriologist sterilizes his smooth platinum needle most carefully in the flame before he uses it for inoculation of an artificial medium, we must realize how much more important it is to sterilize in a most scrupulous manner rough instruments, such as broaches, so as not to inoculate the human tissue. All root-canal instruments should be immersed in alcohol, or in phenol first and alcohol secondly, each time before they are used. The field of operation should be properly prepared by use of

---

* CALAHAN, J. R.: Resin Solution in Root Canals. *Items of Interest*, August, 1915, p. 579.

rubber-dam and scrubbing of the projecting teeth with 10% formaldehyde, which is dried off by means of air. If cotton dressings are used for root canal work, or if broaches wound with cotton are used, a number properly prepared and sterilized should be kept on hand. The cavity should be most carefully sealed after each treatment to keep saliva from entering.

SUMMARY OF IMPORTANT FACTORS TO PREVENT PERIAPICAL INFECTION

The important factors which should be borne in mind in operations of pulp removal, root-canal work and filling, are, in short, the following:

1. Diagnose the condition first by means of a radiograph.

2. Treat only cases which promise a good result.

3. Observe strict aseptic precautions.

4. Extirpate all pulp tissue.

5. Avoid injury and necrosis of the periapical tissue as caused by the use of certain irritating drugs.

6. Avoid infecting of the periapical tissue by instrumentation.

7. If a root canal does not yield treatment in a short time and no radiograph was taken in the first place, take one now with an indicator in the root canal and find out what is wrong.

8. Fill the root canals to the very end and ensure a successful operation by means of another radiograph.

Prevention of Devitalized Teeth.

DEVITALIZATION FOR SENSITIVE DENTINE AND PROSTHESES NOT JUSTIFIED

Our knowledge of the etiology and complications of alveolar abscesses and realization of the uncertainty of root-canal fillings should impress in our minds the seriousness of pulp extirpation. He who extirpates the pulp of one, two or more teeth to restore masticating efficiency by bridge work renders poor services if granulomata develop on the devitalized teeth, which are apt to endanger the patient's health. A pulp for such or similar purposes should not be sacrificed except after the most careful consideration and prognostic study of the roots and root canals by means of radiographs. Prosthetic appliances should be constructed which do not require devitalization of healthy teeth, and our efforts should be in the direction of devising reconstruction work which is not destructive to the remaining hard or soft tissues of the mouth.

TREATMENT OF HYPEREMIA AND EXPOSURES OF THE PULP TO PREVENT DEVITALIZATION Hyperemia and exposures are frequently brought about when excavating cavities if insufficient attention is paid to the approach to the pulp. The pulp horns are especially liable to become accidentally involved. Large metal fillings are liable to cause hyperemia because they are good conductors of heat and cold. A nonconductor should be placed into the deepest parts of the cavity beneath the filling. A pulp in the state of active hyperemia can almost always be saved if the irritating causes are removed. The mildest anodines should be applied, such as oil of cloves or modified phenol slightly warmed, until the irritation has subsided, when the same treatment as for pulp capping is indicated. Pulp capping is performed over deep decayed areas which reach very close to the pulp, and where there is danger of making an exposure if excavation is continued. The action then is that of preservation. In actual small exposures made by excavators in fully formed teeth in cases where the pulp has previously given no symptoms of inflammation, and in exposures of teeth the apical foramen of which is wide open, with pulp normal or very slightly inflamed, we may attempt to save the pulp by the so-called capping method. The patient, however, should be informed of the doubtful outcome of the undertaking. If there is slight hyperemia of the pulp, an anodine such as modified phenol or oil of cloves should first be applied, sealing it into the tooth with quicksetting cement (not gutta percha) for one week. At the second visit zinc oxide and eugenol, mixed to a thin paste, is slightly coaxed over the exposed area; this is covered with a layer of quick-setting cement. All depends upon perfect asepsis, skillful manipulation and prevention of any pressure or irritation. A temporary filling may be used until the result is made sure of.

EARLY TREAT-MENT OF CARIES AND PROPHYLAXIS The prevention of hyperemia, which leads to other diseases of the pulp, is best accomplished by filling the cavities when small and shallow, or better still, in controlling decay by prophylactic treatment. This is also prevention in the highest degree against alveolar abscesses and its many and dangerous complications. The teaching to the public of oral hygiene, which first was principally undertaken to combat the loss of masticating efficiency and its sequels, poor digestion, and ill-health, has now grown to a still greater importance, namely: the prevention of systemic diseases of the gravest nature to which the unsuspecting individual is liable to fall prey. With this point in view, the dentist should educate the public to the far-reaching meaning of preventive dentistry, and offer his patients prophylactic treatment at such intervals as seem necessary for each individual case, and teach each individual how to keep the teeth in good condition by suggestions as to a suitable diet and practical demonstrations of how to take care of teeth and gums at home.

PLATE LXXVIII

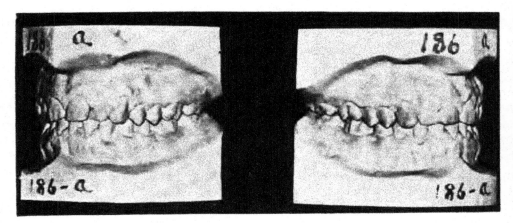

FIG. 286   FIG. 287

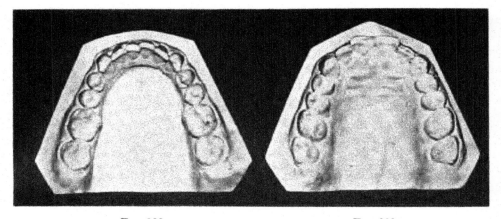

FIG. 288   FIG. 289

FIGS. 286, 287, 288 and 289.—Left and right side view and occlusial view of upper and lower jaw of a patient's teeth who had the four first molars extracted when sixteen years of age. The four illustrations show the condition when the patient was thirty-five years of age.

Reproduced by the courtesy of Dr. Eugene H. Smith.

CHAPTER XII

THE TRUE VALUE OF A TOOTH

Dean Smith, of Harvard University Dental School, in his timely paper read before the First District Dental Society of the State of New York, said: "We all know how difficult it is to adjust material values. How much more difficult it is to adjust physiological values, in the misjudging of which the happiness, health, and frequently the life of the people is jeopardized!" It is indeed difficult to place the right value on a tooth; the judgment depends a good deal on education, education of the dentist and education of his patients. The value of a healthy tooth in good occlusion is the easier to determine; it certainly cannot be overestimated, but if a tooth is affected by any of the various dental diseases, there arises a great difference of opinion. Among the various pathological conditions I shall consider only those we are especially concerned with in this book, namely, the oral abscesses and systemic diseases which are caused by them. One cannot place too low a value on a devitalized tooth if it causes conditions which endanger the patient's health.

The tooth which is the most frequent cause of abscesses is the first permanent molar. This tooth, which plays such an important part in the health, decays under our very eyes in children who have the best of care, unless the fissures are carefully filled as soon as the gum has shrunken away from the occlusial surface. In the poor, who do not care for their teeth except if so forced by pain, this tooth is almost always a ruin when it comes under our observation, and its pulp is invariably diseased and very often periapical infection has already set in. The value of this tooth sinks then from the highest mark to

the lowest level. Such badly decayed teeth are continuous expenses, as they would have to be filled and refilled
and finally crowned, and would be sure, sooner or later,
to cause periapical infection. The poison which discharges into the system from such a focus only lowers
the child's resistance to various illnesses, and hampers
the development of the body, but, worse than all, may
cause systemic diseases of the gravest nature from which
recovery may be impossible. How much better is extraction in such cases; the twelve-year molars will move forward into place, and while it would not always result in an
ideal condition, the condition which the orthodontist calls
"perfect occlusion," it would, if symmetrically carried
out, be just as good as what the average person has; per-
sonally, I would say infinitely better, because a first molar
with periapical infection would have to be extracted
sooner or later; it is only a matter of time; and when extracted in later life it will leave a space which cannot then
be filled in by nature, the second molars having been firmly
fixed in the bone at that period of life; for the patient the
result is worse from any point of view: that of occlusion,
masticating efficiency, chance of systemic infection, and
loss of time and money.

The saving of teeth in children should be of preventive
nature, which is the only safe way of securing and keep-
ing normal occlusion; but if it is too late for prevention,
we must be satisfied with the next best healthy condition.
The results obtained from symmetric extraction of the
badly decayed permanent first molars are very satisfactory if undertaken before the age of twelve; the occlusion
is in the majority of cases very good, as has been named
"sufficient occlusion" by Dean Smith, a term which expresses the condition fully. Figures 286 to 293 show
models of two patients who had the first permanent molars
extracted at the proper age on account of extensive decay,
and the results are gratifying. These illustrations have
been reproduced with Dr. Smith's consent from his
already mentioned paper. While I want it clearly understood that I do not believe in the wholesale extraction of

PLATE LXXIX

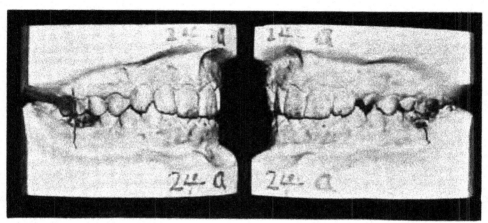

FIG. 290   FIG. 291

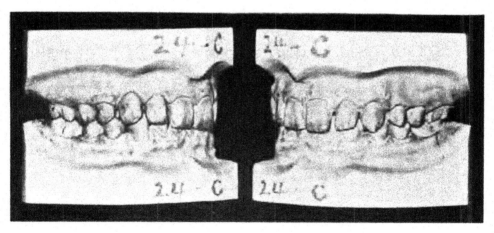

FIG. 292   FIG. 293

FIGS. 290 and 291.—Left and right view of the teeth of a boy aged thirteen. The right lower first molar is half decayed, pulp involved, apical foramina open. The left lower first molar has an exposed pulp. The upper first molars are decayed. All the first molars were extracted, no appliances had been used and already after three years the good result shown in Figs. 292 and 293 were obtained.

Reproduced by the courtesy of Dr. Eugene H. Smith.

children's teeth, and that neither Dr. Smith nor I would advise the above treatment except in cases where the first molars are in hopeless condition, I would say this: that I for one should much prefer to own any of the mouths shown in these pictures with only "sufficient occlusion" of twenty-eight healthy teeth, than an ideal occlusion with a number of devitalized teeth and arthritic joints.

The value of healthy teeth is so inestimably high that every effort should be made to preserve them. A devitalized tooth diminishes greatly in value if an abscess is formed at its roots, but when it becomes a focus of ill-health and disease in other parts of the body, its value becomes decidedly negative and its ownership a curse.

BIBLIOGRAPHY

ADAMI & McCRAE, Textbook of Pathology. (Lea & Ferbiger, Philadelphia.)

ADLOFF, P. Zur Frage der Herkunft des Epithels in den Wurzelsystem. (see Deutsche Monatsschr. f. Zahnheilkunde.)

BAEHR, G. Glomerular Lesions of Subacute Bacterial Endocarditis. (see Journal of Experimental Medicine, Vol. 15.)

BECK, J. C. Chronic Focal Infection of the Nose, Throat, Mouth and Ear. (see Journal of American Medical Association, November, 1914, Vol. LXIII, p. 1636.)

BELLEI, G. A Short Contribution to the Study of General Infection produced by Staphylococcus Aureus and by the Steptococcus. (see Lancet, March, 1902.)

BERGER, A. Dento Alveolar Abscess. (see Items of Interest, September, 1914, p. 641.)

BILLINGS, F. Clinical Aspect and Medical Management of Arthritis Deformans. (see Illinois Medical Journal, January, 1914.)
    The Medical Management of Chronic Arthritis. (see Illinois Medical Journal, September, 1914.)
    Focal Infection. (see Journal of American Medical Association, September, 1914, V. LXIII, p. 899.)
    Chronic Focal Infections as a Causative Factor in Chronic Arthritis. (see Journal of American Medical Association, September, 1913, Vol. LXI, p. 819.)
    Mouth Infection as a Source of Systemic Disease. (see Journal of American Medical Association, December, 1914.)

BRAMWELL, B. Notes on the Treatment of Pernicious Anemia. (British Medical Journal, January, 1909, p. 209.)

BROPHY, T. W. Oral Surgery. (P. Blakiston's Son & Co.)

BUNTING, R. W. The Pathology of the Dental Pulp. (see Dental Cosmos, February, 1915, p. 143.)

BUSH, B. E. The Close Relation of the Dentist and the Physician. (Journal American Medical Association, 1910, p. 752.)

BUTT, WM. REDFIELD. Nose, Throat and Ear as Neighboring Organs to the Teeth. (see The Dental Cosmos, August, 1915, p. 837.)

CABOT, R. C. Analysis of Six Hundred Cases of Heart Disease. (*Journal of the American Medical Association*, 1914, Vol. IXIII.)

CALLAHAN, J. R. Root Canal Preparation. (*see Items of Interest*, August, 1915, p. 567.)

CAMAC, C. N. B. Dental Sepsis: Its Relation to the System. (*see Journal of the National Dental Association*, November, 1915, p. 8.)

CANTANI, PROF. ARNALDO. La Clinica Italiana. June and July, 1914.

CARABELLI, G. Elden von Lunkaszprie, Anatomie des Mundes. Wien, 1842.

CAVEN, W. P. The Importance of Oral and Dental Conditions. (*Dominion Dental Journal*, 1912.)

COLYER, J. F. Oral Sepsis and its Relation to General Diseases. (*Journal British Dental Association*, Vol. XXIII, p. 409.)

COLYER, J. & S. Dental Disease in its Relation to General Medicine. (London: Longman's, 1911.)

CORWIN, J. W. Fetid Breath. (*see Items of Interest*, November, 1914, p. 827; also discussion, p. 855.)

CRAIG, C. BURNS. Periodontal Infection as a Causative Factor in Nervous Diseases. (*see Journal of the American Medical Association*, December 5, 1914.)

DALTON. A Case Showing Relationship to Oral Sepsis. (*British Medical Journal*, November, 1914, p. 1368.)

DALY, R. R. Relations of Dental and Rhinologic Work. (*see Dental Cosmos, January*, 1915, p. 43.)

DAVIS, D. J. Bacteriology and Pathology of the Tonsils with Especial Reference to Chronic Articular, Renal and Cardiac Lesions. (*see Journal of Infectious Diseases*, Vol. X, No. 2, March, 1912, p. 148.)

DAVIS, WM. T. The Inter-relation of the Teeth and the Eye. (*see The Dental Cosmos*, July, 1915, p. 769.)

DEPENDORP, TH. Zur Pathogenese der Zahnwurzelzyzstem. (*see Deutsche Monatsschr. f. Zahnheilkunde*, November, 1912, p. 809.)

DE VECCHIS, B. New Problems Regarding Tubercular Infection and a Special Treatment for Cervical Adenitis following Oral Sepsis. (*see Dental Cosmos*, July, 1915, p. 737.)

DORRANCE, GEORGE MORRIS. Enlarged Cervical Glands, with Special Reference to the Mouth as an Etiological Factor. (*see The Dental Cosmos*, August, 1913, p. 808.)

DOXTATER, L. W. Constitutional Infection due to Chronic Dento-Alveolar Abscess and Pyorrhoea Alveolaris. (*see Dental Cosmos*, September, 1915, p. 983.)

DRESCHFIELD, H. T. Dental Diseases and their Relation to Public Health. (*Journal of London Institution*, Vol. XXIII, 1903, p. 867.)

EDITORIAL. Mouth Infection and Systemic Disease. (*see Items of Interest*, December, 1915, p. 943.)

EISEN, E. J. & IVY R. H. Origin and Metastatic Importance of Chronic Oral Infections. (*see Items of Interest*, February, 1916, p. 81.)

EUSTIS, R. S. Endocarditis in Children. (*see Boston Medical and Surgical Journal*, September, 1915, p. 348.)

FEILER, BRESLAU. Zur Anatomie des Foramen Apicale. (*Deutsche Monatsschr. f. Zahnheilkunde.*)

GILBERTI. Medical Practice Series, 1910, V. III, p. 313.)

GILDERSLEEVE, NATH. Oral Infections. (*see The Dental Cosmos*, December, 1915, p. 1350.)

GILLETT, HENRY W. Management of Badly Mutilated Mouths. (*see Journal of Allied Dental Societies*, December, 1915, p. 431.)

GILMER, J. L. Chronic Oral Infections. (*see Archives of Internal Medicine*, April, 1912, Vol. 9, p. 499.)

GILMER, J. L. and MOODY, A. M. A Study of the Bacteriology of Alveolar Abscess and Infected Root Canals. (*see Journal of American Medical Association*, December, 1914, Vol. LXIII, p. 2023.)

GOLDTHWAIT, PAINTER & OSGOOD. Diseases of the Bones and Joints. (Boston: D. C. Heath & Co.)

GRAYSON, C. P. The Teeth in Relation to Ear and Throat Diseases. (*see The Dental Cosmos*, June, 1907, p. 555.)

GRIEVES, C. J. Systemic Pus Poisoning Associated with Diseased Dental Apical Regions. (*see Items of Interest*, May, 1911, p. 339.)

Dental Periapical Infections as the Cause of Systemic Disease. (*see The Dental Cosmos*, January, 1914, p. 52.)

Unhygienic Mouths. (*see The Dental Cosmos*, November, 1913, p. 1102.)

The Responsibilities of the Dentist in Systemic Diseases Arising from Dento-Alveolar Abscess as Illustrated by the Etiology of Periodontal Abscess. (*see Dental Cosmos*, May 1914, p. 564.)

GRIEVES C. J.—*Continued.*

Secondary Infections. (*see Journal of Allied Dental Societies*, June, 1914, p. 178.)

The Relation of the Vitality of the Periapical Cementum and Adjacent Tissues to the Patient's Health, and the Status of the Dental Profession. (*see The Dental Cosmos,* October, 1915, p. 1112.)

Artificial Production of Apical Necrosis by Root Canal Drugging. (*see The Dental Cosmos,* October, 1915, p. 1119.)

HAMANN, C. A. Some of the Complications and Results of Dental Infections. (*see Wisconsin Medical Journal,* March, 1903.)

HARTZEL, T. B. Two Preliminary Reports of Arthritis Caused by Dental Abscess. (*see* Official Bulletin of National Dental Association, March, 1914, p. 4.)

Report of the Minnesota Division of the Scientific Foundation and Research Commission. (*see Journal of National Dental Association,* November, 1915, p. 333.)

The Clinical Type of Arthritis Originating about the Teeth. (*see Journal of American Medical Association,* September, 1915, p. 1093.)

Secondary Infections having their Primary Origin in the Oral Cavity. (*see Journal of Allied Dental Societies,* June, 1914, p. 166.)

Report: Mouth Infection Research Corps of National Dental Association. (*see* Official Bulletin, National Dental Association, October, 1914, p. 48.)

HUNTER, WILLIAM. Pernicious Anaemia. (London: Charles Griffin & Co., Ltd.)

HUSCHART, J. H. The Relation Diseases of the Teeth Bear to the Eye and Ear. (*see Dental Brief,* Vol. XII, p. 799.)

IDMANN, GÖSTA. Bakteriologische Untersuchungen von periostalen Abszessen (*see Arbeiten aus dem Pathologischen Institut der Universität Helsingfors,* Erster Band, Gustav Fischer, Jena, 1913.)

JONES, W. I. Treatment of Impacted Third Molars. (*see Items of Interest,* October, 1915, p. 786.)

KAUFFMANN, JOSEPH HERBERT. Abscess and Pyemia? A Case of Extensive Alveolar Abscess Associated with Pyemia. (*see The Dental Cosmos,* May, 1915, p. 530.)

KRAUSE, HEYMANN. Lehrbuch der chirurgischen Operationen. (Urban & Schwarzenberg, Berlin, Wien.)

LANGWORTHY, HENRY GLOVER. Some Remarks on the Removal of Troublesome Tonsils of Interest to Dentists. (*see The Dental Cosmos,* July, 1913, p. 718.)

LAWRENCE, CHAS. H. Chronic Arthritis. (Paper read before the Boston Surgical Fortnightly Club, October, 1915.)

LEE, R. I. Preventable Heart Disease. (see Boston Medical and Surgical Journal, July, 1915, p. 157.)

LEHMANN, K. B. & NEUMANN, R. O. Bakteriologie und Bakteriologische Diagnose. (München, 1907: Verlag von I. I. Lehmann.)

LEVER, J. W. Pneumococcic Arthritis with Report of Six Cases. (see Boston Medical and Surgical Journal, September, 1915, p. 387.)

LEVY, M., Berlin. Statistische Untersuchungen über den Zusammenhang von Zahnkaries und Rheumatismus und Gicht. (Deutsche Monatsschr. für Zahnheilkunde, June, 1914, p. 436.)

LOGAN, W. H. G. Blood Findings in 162 Consecutive Cases of Chronic Oral Infection Associated with Teeth. (see Items of Interest, December, 1915, p. 912.)

LYONS, C. J. The Pathological Significance of Impacted and Unerupted Teeth. (see The Journal of the National Dental Association, March, 1916, p. 28.)

MACKEE, G. M. and REMER, JOHN. Oral Sepsis as a Focus of Infection. (see American Journal of Roentgenology, p. 158.)

MALLORY, FRANK B. Principles of Pathologic Histology. W. B. Saunders Co.

MAY, CHARLES H. Manual of Diseases of the Eye. (William Wood & Co., New York.)

MAYO, C. H. Mouth Infection as a Source of Systemic Disease. (see Journal of American Medical Association, December, 1914, Vol. LXIII, p. 2025.)

MEDALIA, LEON S. The Use of Bacterial Vaccines in Acute Septic Conditions of the Oral Cavity met with by the Dentist, with Special Reference to Mandibular and Septic Apical Abscesses. (see The Dental Cosmos, January, 1914, p. 12.)

MEX, P. Beobachtungen über den Zusammenhang periodontitischen Erkrankungen zu Allgemeinkrankheiten, insbesondere zu den Drüsenerkrankungen der Kinder. (Deutsche Monatsschr. f. Zahnheilkunde, March, 1913.)

MILNE, L. S. Chronic Arthritis. (see Journal of American Medical Association, February, 1914, Vol. LXII, p. 593.)

MINER, L. M. S. Antagonistic Therapy: Its Laboratory Aspects and Its Application in Septic Processes of the Oral Cavity. (see Journal of Allied Societies, March, 1910.)

MONIER. Contribution à l'étude pathologique des infections dentaires. Thèse de Paris, 1914. (Steinheil.)

NEUMANN, R., Berlin. Die Wurzelspitzenresektion an den unteren Molaren. Verlag von Hermann Meusser.

NODINE, A. M. Rheumatic Fever and the Contribution of a Septic Mouth and Carious Teeth to its Cause and Cure. (*see Items of Interest*, September, 1912, p. 656.)

ORTON, F. H. Root Canal Filling. (*see Items of Interest*, November, 1915, p. 801.)

OSLER, SIR WILLIAM. The Principles and Practice of Medicine. (D. Appleton & Co., London.)

PARK, WILLIAM HALLOCK, and WILLIAMS, ANNA W. Pathogenic Microörganisms. (New York: Lea & Febiger.)

PARTSCH. Die Chronische Wurzelhautentzündung. (*Deutsche Zahneilkunde in Vorträgen*, Leipzig.)

PERKINS, A. F. Root Canals Which Cannot be Filled. (*see Items of Interest*, November, 1915, p. 806.)

PHILLIPS, W. CHARLES. Diseases of the Ear, Nose and Throat. (Philadelphia, 1911.)

PREISWERK, GUSTAV. Zahnheilkunde, J. F. Lehmann. München, 1908.

PROELL. Weiteres zur Mikroskopie der Granulome und Zahnwurzelzystem. (*Deutsche Montsschr. f. Zahnheilkunde*, January, 1913, p. 1.)
    Über die Mikroskopie der Granulome, Entstehung und Wachstum der Zahnwurzelzystem. (*Deutsche Monatsschr. f. Zahnheilkunde*, July, 1911, p. 558.)
    Zur Mikroskopie der Granulome und Zahnwurzelzystem. (*Deutsche Monatsschr. f. Zahnheilkunde*, March, 1911, p. 161.)

RAPER, H. R. Bad Canal Work. What Shall We Do About It? (*see Dental Items of Interest*, February, 1916, p. 111.)

RHEIN, M. L. The Dental Aspect of Oral Infection. (*see Items of Interest*, June, 1914, p. 439.)
    Infected Areas Around the Ends of Roots of Teeth. (*see Journal of American Medical Association*, August, 1912, Vol. LIX., p. 361.)
    Scientific Treatment of Root Canals. (*see Dental Cosmos*, September, 1911.)
    Deep-seated Alveolar Infections. (*see Surgery, Gynecology and Obstetrics*, January, 1916, p. 33.)

ROE, W. J. Surgical Lesions Due to Oral Sepsis and Their Treatment. (*see The Dental Cosmos*, February, 1915, p. 174.)

ROSENOW, E. C. Lesions Produced by Various Streptococci, Endocarditis, and Rheumatism. (see *New York Medical Journal*, February, 1914, p. 270.)

The Production of Ulcer of the Stomach by Injection of Streptococci. (see *Journal of American Medical Association*, November, 1913, Vol. LXI, p. 1947.)

The Newer Bacteriology of Various Infections as Determined by Special Methods. (see *Journal of American Medical Association*, September, 1914, p. 903.)

Mouth Infection as a Source of Systemic Disease. (see *Journal of American Medical Association*, December, 1914.)

Transmutations within the Streptococcus Pneumococcus Group. (see *Journal of Infectious Diseases*, Vol. 14, January, 1914.)

The Etiology of Acute Rheumatism, Articular and Muscular. (see *Journal of Infectious Diseases*, Vol. 14, January, 1914.)

RUMPEL, C. Die Plasmazellen des Zahngranuloms. (see *Vierteljahrsschrift für Zahnheilkunde*, January, 1911, p. 60.)

SAWYER, A. J. Oral Sepsis as the Cause of General or Systemic Infection, and the Dentist's Responsibility. (see *The Dental Cosmos*, March, 1915, p. 272.)

SCHAMBERG, M. I. Dentistry, a Blessing and a Curse. (see *Journal of Allied Dental Association*, December, 1915, p. 418.)

SCHUSTER, ERNST. Die Sektion der Zahnwurzel eine Operationsmethode zur Entfernung abgebrochener Instrumente aus Wurzelkanälen. (*Deutsche Monatsschr. für Zahnheilkunde*, January, 1913, p. 43.)

SCHWABE. Beziehungen zwischen Augen und Zahnkkrankheiten. (*Deutsche Monatsschr. für Zahnheilkunde*, June, 1914, p. 401.)

SMITH, A. H. Some Studies of the Jaws in Health and Disease. (see *The Dental Cosmos*, August, 1913, p. 765.)

SMITH, E. H. The Value of a Tooth. (see *The Journal of Allied Dental Societies*, September, 1915, p. 331.)

STEINHARTER, E. C. Gastric Ulcer Experimentally Produced. (*Boston Medical and Surgical Journal*, May 11, 1916.)

Acute Arthritis Experimentally Produced by Intravenous Injection of the Staphylococcus Pyogenes. (*Boston Medical and Surgical Journal*, July 13, 1916.)

STORCK, J. A. Teeth as a Factor in Digestive Diseases and Disorders. (see *New Orleans Medical and Surgical Journal*, January, 1904, p. 497.)

STRAUSSBERG, M. Successful Treatment of Apical Abscesses by Ionization. (see *Dental Items of Interest*, April, 1915, p. 259.)

STREITMANN, W. H.   Oral Sepsis as Related to Systemic Disease. (see *Items of Interest,* December, 1915, p. 930.)

STURRIDGE, ERNEST.   Dental Electro Therapeutics.   (Philadelphia: Lea & Febiger.)

TEAGUE, B. H.   The Recognition of Systemic Disturbance in the Treatment of Oral Lesions.   (see *The Dental Cosmos,* April, 1915, p. 428.)

THOMA, KURT H.   Oral Anaesthesia.   (Boston: Ritter & Flebbe.)
Oral Anaesthesia with Special Reference to Surgical Operations for Chronic Alveolar Abscesses. (see *American Journal of Surgery,* Vol. I, No. 3, April, 1915.)
Oral Abscesses.   (see *Journal of the Allied Dental Societies,* March, 1916.)

THOMAS, J. D.   The Effects of Prolonged Treatment and Persistent Retention of Diseased Teeth.   (see *Items of Interest,* August 1912, p. 617.)

THOMSON, SIR ST. CLAIR.   Diseases of the Nose and Throat.   (London: D. Appleton & Co.)

ULRICH, H. L.   Streptococcicosis.   (see *Journal-Lancet,* November, 1915.)
The Blind Dental Abscess.   (see *Journal of American Medical Association,* November, 1915, Vol. LXV, p. 1619.)
Some Medical Aspects of Certain Mouth Infections.   (see *Dental Review,* December, 1914.)

VAN DOORN, J. W.   Relation of Dental Lesions to Insomnia and Nerve Strain.   (see *The Dental Cosmos,* June, 1909, p. 677.)

VAUGHAN, V. C.   Die Phänomena der Infektion und Ergebuisse der Immunitätsforschung Experimentellen Therapie, Bakteriologie und Hygiene.   (see *Fortsetzung des Jahresberichts über die Ergebuisse der Immunitätsforschung.*)

VAUGHAN, WALTER, VICTOR C., and VICTOR C., JR.   Protein Split Products in Relation to Immunity and Disease.   (Lea & Febiger.)

WALLACE, J. SIM, London.   Dental Diseases in Relation to Public Health.   (Publishing Office of *The Dental Record,* 1914.) (*Deutsche Monatsschr. für Zahnheilkunde,* June, 1914.)

WILLIGER, FRITZ.   Zahnärztliche Chirurgie, Berlin.   (Leitfaden der Praktischen Medizen, Band I, 1910.)

YOUNG, J. H.   Tonsillectomy as a Therapeutic Measure in the Treatment of Chorea and Endocarditis.   (see *Boston Medical and Surgical Journal,* September, 1915, p. 356.)

ZILZ, JULJAN.   Zur Klinik und Pathologischen Anatomie der Speichelsteine.   (see *Zeitschrift für Mund-und Kierferchirurgie und Greuzgebiete,* Erster Band, Erstes Heft, p. 32.)

INDEX OF ILLUSTRATIONS

INDEX